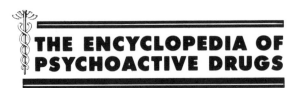

# THE ENCYCLOPEDIA OF PSYCHOACTIVE DRUGS

## SERIES 1

The Addictive Personality
Alcohol and Alcoholism
Alcohol Customs and Rituals
Alcohol Teenage Drinking
Amphetamines Danger in the Fast Lane
Barbiturates Sleeping Potion or Intoxicant?
Caffeine The Most Popular Stimulant
Cocaine A New Epidemic
Escape from Anxiety and Stress
Flowering Plants Magic in Bloom
Getting Help Treatments for Drug Abuse
Heroin The Street Narcotic
Inhalants The Toxic Fumes

LSD Visions or Nightmares?
Marijuana Its Effects on Mind & Body
Methadone Treatment for Addiction
Mushrooms Psychedelic Fungi
Nicotine An Old-Fashioned Addiction
Over-The-Counter Drugs Harmless or Hazardous?
PCP The Dangerous Angel
Prescription Narcotics The Addictive Painkillers
Quaaludes The Quest for Oblivion
Teenage Depression and Drugs
Treating Mental Illness
Valium ® and Other Tranquilizers

## SERIES 2

Bad Trips
Brain Function
Case Histories
Celebrity Drug Use
Designer Drugs
The Downside of Drugs
Drinking, Driving, and Drugs
Drugs and Civilization
Drugs and Crime
Drugs and Diet
Drugs and Disease
Drugs and Emotion
Drugs and Pain
Drugs and Perception
Drugs and Pregnancy
Drugs and Sexual Behavior

Drugs and Sleep
Drugs and Sports
Drugs and the Arts
Drugs and the Brain
Drugs and the Family
Drugs and the Law
Drugs and Women
Drugs of the Future
Drugs Through the Ages
Drug Use Around the World
Legalization A Debate
Mental Disturbances
Nutrition and the Brain
The Origins and Sources of Drugs
Substance Abuse Prevention and Cures
Who Uses Drugs?

# MENTAL
# DISTURBANCES

GENERAL EDITOR
Professor Solomon H. Snyder, M.D.
*Distinguished Service Professor of
Neuroscience, Pharmacology, and Psychiatry at
The Johns Hopkins University School of Medicine*

•

ASSOCIATE EDITOR
Professor Barry L. Jacobs, Ph.D.
*Program in Neuroscience, Department of Psychology,
Princeton University*

•

SENIOR EDITORIAL CONSULTANT
Joann Rodgers
*Deputy Director, Office of Public Affairs at
The Johns Hopkins Medical Institutions*

*l*

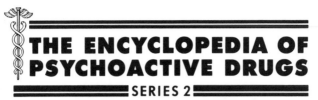

# THE ENCYCLOPEDIA OF PSYCHOACTIVE DRUGS
## SERIES 2

# MENTAL DISTURBANCES

PATRICK YOUNG

**CHELSEA HOUSE PUBLISHERS**
NEW YORK • NEW HAVEN • PHILADELPHIA

EDITOR-IN-CHIEF: Nancy Toff
EXECUTIVE EDITOR: Remmel T. Nunn
MANAGING EDITOR: Karyn Gullen Browne
COPY CHIEF: Juliann Barbato
PICTURE EDITOR: Adrian G. Allen
ART DIRECTOR: Giannella Garrett
MANUFACTURING MANAGER: Gerald Levine

*Staff for* MENTAL DISTURBANCES:

SENIOR EDITOR: Jane Larkin Crain
ASSOCIATE EDITOR: Paula Edelson
ASSISTANT EDITOR: Laura-Ann Dolce
COPY EDITOR: Ellen Scordato
EDITORIAL ASSISTANT: Susan DeRosa
ASSOCIATE PICTURE EDITOR: Juliette Dickstein
PICTURE RESEARCHER: Debra P. Hershkowitz
DESIGNER: Victoria Tomaselli
DESIGN ASSISTANT: Donna Sinisgalli
PRODUCTION COORDINATOR: Joseph Romano
COVER ILLUSTRATION: *Volto Grottesco* by Leonardo da Vinci

CREATIVE DIRECTOR: Harold Steinberg

Library of Congress Cataloging in Publication Data

Young, Patrick.
    Mental Disturbances.
    (Encyclopedia of psychoactive drugs. Series 2)
    Bibliography: p.
    Includes index.
    1. Mental illness—Juvenile literature. 2. Drugs—Toxicology—Juvenile
literature. 3. Psychopharmacology—Juvenile literature. [1. Mental illness. 2.
Drugs]
    I. Title. II. Series. [DNLM: 1. Drugs—adverse effects—popular works. 2.
Mental Disorders—popular works. WM 75 Y75m]
RC460.2.Y68   1988      616.89      87-25688

ISBN 1-55546-206-5

# CONTENTS

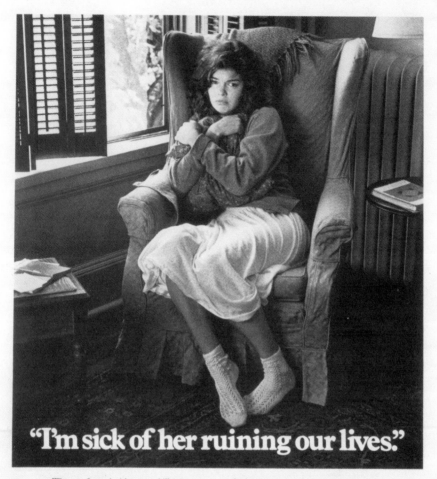

## "I'm sick of her ruining our lives."

When confronted with a mental illness, many families experience a wide range of confusing and upsetting emotions. From outrage to despair, shame and denial.

They often blame victims for causing worry, embarrassment, family strife. And they can often blame themselves. "Was it my fault?" "Where did I go wrong?"

But, mental illness is no one's fault. Least of all those afflicted. It's a serious medical illness that affects one in four families—afflicting 35 million Americans from all walks of life.

Recognizing the warning signs and seeking professional treatment for your loved one can be the first steps to reducing family fears and confusion. And to actually healing the sickness.

Today, mental illness need not be hopeless. Due to recent progress in research and treatment, two out of three victims can get better and lead productive lives.

But they can't do it alone. They need your compassion, support, and understanding.

Learn more. For an informative booklet, write: The American Mental Health Fund, P.O. Box 17700, Washington, D.C. 20041. Or call toll free: 1-800-433-5959. In Illinois, call: 1-800-826-2336.

 **Learn to see the sickness. Learning is the key to healing.**

THE AMERICAN MENTAL HEALTH FUND

---

*A poster highlights the emotional assault mental illness wages on its victims and their families. Fortunately, many diseases of the mind can now be treated with psychotherapy and psychiatric drugs.*

# In the Mainstream
# of American Life

One of the legacies of the social upheaval of the 1960s is that psychoactive drugs have become part of the mainstream of American life. Schools, homes, and communities cannot be "drug proofed." There is a demand for drugs — and the supply is plentiful. Social norms have changed and drugs are not only available—they are everywhere.

But where efforts to curtail the supply of drugs and outlaw their use have had tragically limited effects on demand, it may be that education has begun to stem the rising tide of drug abuse among young people and adults alike.

Over the past 25 years, as drugs have become an increasingly routine facet of contemporary life, a great many teenagers have adopted the notion that drug taking was somehow a right or a privilege or a necessity. They have done so, however, without understanding the consequences of drug use during the crucial years of adolescence.

The teenage years are few in the total life cycle, but critical in the maturation process. During these years adolescents face the difficult tasks of discovering their identity, clarifying their sexual roles, asserting their independence, learning to cope with authority, and searching for goals that will give their lives meaning.

Drugs rob adolescents of precious time, stamina, and health. They interrupt critical learning processes, sometimes forever. Teenagers who use drugs are likely to withdraw increasingly into themselves, to "cop out" at just the time when they most need to reach out and experience the world.

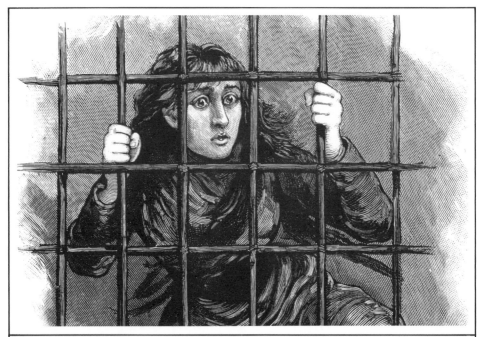

*An 1882 woodcut of an insane woman behind bars. Even in the more enlightened 1980s, the mentally ill are subjected to fear and ridicule.*

Fortunately, as a recent Gallup poll shows, young people are beginning to realize this, too. They themselves label drugs their most important problem. In the last few years, moreover, the climate of tolerance and ignorance surrounding drugs has been changing.

Adolescents as well as adults are becoming aware of mounting evidence that every race, ethnic group, and class is vulnerable to drug dependency.

Recent publicity about the cost and failure of drug rehabilitation efforts; dangerous drug use among pilots, air traffic controllers, star athletes, and Hollywood celebrities; and drug-related accidents, suicides, and violent crime have focused the public's attention on the need to wage an all-out war on drug abuse before it seriously undermines the fabric of society itself.

The anti-drug message is getting stronger and there is evidence that the message is beginning to get through to adults and teenagers alike.

war on drug abuse before it seriously undermines the fabric of society itself.

The anti-drug message is getting stronger and there is evidence that the message is beginning to get through to adults and teenagers alike.

*The Encyclopedia of Psychoactive Drugs* hopes to play a part in the national campaign now underway to educate young people about drugs. Series 1 provides clear and comprehensive discussions of common psychoactive substances, outlines their psychological and physiological effects on the mind and body, explains how they "hook" the user, and separates fact from myth in the complex issue of drug abuse.

Whereas Series 1 focuses on specific drugs, such as nicotine or cocaine, Series 2 confronts a broad range of both social and physiological phenomena. Each volume addresses the ramifications of drug use and abuse on some aspect of human experience: social, familial, cultural, historical, and physical. Separate volumes explore questions about the effects of drugs on brain chemistry and unborn children; the use and abuse of painkillers; the relationship between drugs and sexual behavior, sports, and the arts; drugs and disease; the role of drugs in history; and the sophisticated drugs now being developed in the laboratory that will profoundly change the future.

Each book in the series is fully illustrated and is tailored to the needs and interests of young readers. The more adolescents know about drugs and their role in society, the less likely they are to misuse them.

Joann Rodgers
*Senior Editorial Consultant*

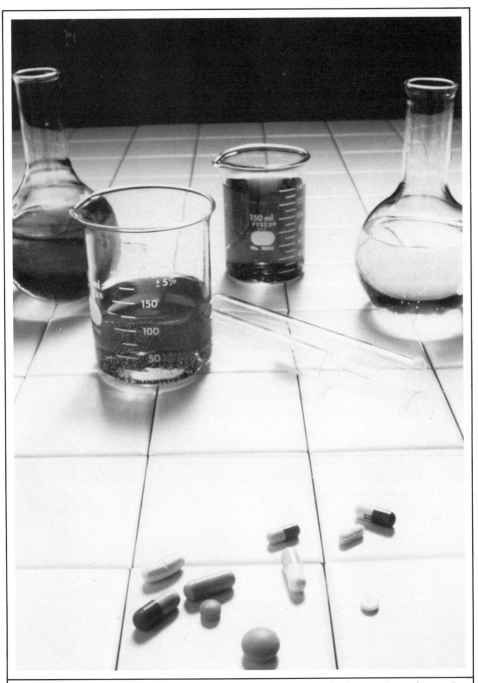

*Research into the chemistry of the brain has revealed the physiological basis of many emotional disturbances. This in turn has lead to the development of specific drugs to treat a variety of these illnesses.*

# INTRODUCTION

## The Gift of Wizardry
## Use and Abuse

**JACK H. MENDELSON, M.D.**
**NANCY K. MELLO, Ph.D.**
*Alcohol and Drug Abuse Research Center*
*Harvard Medical School—McLean Hospital*

Dorothy to the Wizard:

"I think you are a very bad man," said Dorothy.
"Oh no, my dear; I'm really a very good man; but I'm a very bad Wizard."
—from THE WIZARD OF OZ

Man is endowed with the gift of wizardry, a talent for discovery and invention. The discovery and invention of substances that change the way we feel and behave are among man's special accomplishments, and, like so many other products of our wizardry, these substances have the capacity to harm as well as to help. Psychoactive drugs can cause profound changes in the chemistry of the brain and other vital organs, and although their legitimate use can relieve pain and cure disease, their abuse leads in a tragic number of cases to destruction.

Consider alcohol — available to all and yet regarded with intense ambivalence from biblical times to the present day. The use of alcoholic beverages dates back to our earliest ancestors. Alcohol use and misuse became associated with the worship of gods and demons. One of the most powerful Greek gods was Dionysus, lord of fruitfulness and god of wine. The Romans adopted Dionysus but changed his name to Bacchus. Festivals and holidays associated with Bacchus celebrated the harvest and the origins of life. Time has blurred the images of the Bacchanalian festival, but the theme of drunkenness as a major part of celebration has survived the pagan gods and remains a familiar part of modern society. The term "Bacchanalian Festival" conveys a more appealing image than "drunken orgy" or "pot party," but whatever the label, drinking alcohol is a form of drug use that results in addiction for millions.

The fact that many millions of other people can use alcohol in moderation does not mitigate the toll this drug takes on society as a whole. According to reliable estimates, one out of every ten Americans develops a serious alcohol-related problem sometime in his or her lifetime. In addition, automobile accidents caused by drunken drivers claim the lives of tens of thousands every year. Many of the victims are gifted young people, just starting out in adult life. Hospital emergency rooms abound with patients seeking help for alcohol-related injuries.

Who is to blame? Can we blame the many manufacturers who produce such an amazing variety of alcoholic beverages? Should we blame the educators who fail to explain the perils of intoxication, or so exaggerate the dangers of drinking that no one could possibly believe them? Are friends to blame — those peers who urge others to "drink more and faster," or the macho types who stress the importance of being able to "hold your liquor"? Casting blame, however, is hardly constructive, and pointing the finger is a fruitless way to deal with the problem. Alcoholism and drug abuse have few culprits but many victims. Accountability begins with each of us, every time we choose to use or misuse an intoxicating substance.

It is ironic that some of man's earliest medicines, derived from natural plant products, are used today to poison and to intoxicate. Relief from pain and suffering is one of society's many continuing goals. Over 3,000 years ago, the Therapeutic Papyrus of Thebes, one of our earliest written records, gave instructions for the use of opium in the treatment of pain. Opium, in the form of its major derivative, morphine, and similar compounds, such as heroin, have also been used by many to induce changes in mood and feeling. Another example of man's misuse of a natural substance is the coca leaf, which for centuries was used by the Indians of Peru to reduce fatigue and hunger. Its modern derivative, cocaine, has important medical use as a local anesthetic. Unfortunately, its increasing abuse in the 1980s clearly has reached epidemic proportions.

The purpose of this series is to explore in depth the psychological and behavioral effects that psychoactive drugs have on the individual, and also, to investigate the ways in which drug use influences the legal, economic, cultural, and even moral aspects of societies. The information presented here (and in other books in this series) is based on many clinical and laboratory studies and other observations by people from diverse walks of life.

Over the centuries, novelists, poets, and dramatists have provided us with many insights into the sometimes seductive but ultimately problematic aspects of alcohol and drug use. Physicians, lawyers, biologists, psychologists, and social scientists have contributed to a better understanding of the causes and consequences of using these substances. The authors in this series have attempted to gather and condense all the latest information about drug use and abuse. They have also described the sometimes wide gaps in our knowledge and have suggested some new ways to answer many difficult questions.

One such question, for example, is how do alcohol and drug problems get started? And what is the best way to treat them when they do? Not too many years ago, alcoholics and drug abusers were regarded as evil, immoral, or both. It is now recognized that these persons suffer from very complicated diseases involving deep psychological and social problems. To understand how the disease begins and progresses, it is necessary to understand the nature of the substance, the behavior of addicts, and the characteristics of the society or culture in which they live.

Although many of the social environments we live in are very similar, some of the most subtle differences can strongly influence our thinking and behavior. Where we live, go to school and work, whom we discuss things with — all influence our opinions about drug use and misuse. Yet we also share certain commonly accepted beliefs that outweigh any differences in our attitudes. The authors in this series have tried to identify and discuss the central, most crucial issues concerning drug use and misuse.

Despite the increasing sophistication of the chemical substances we create in the laboratory, we have a long way to go in our efforts to make these powerful drugs work for us rather than against us.

The volumes in this series address a wide range of timely questions. What influence has drug use had on the arts? Why do so many of today's celebrities and star athletes use drugs, and what is being done to solve this problem? What is the relationship between drugs and crime? What is the physiological basis for the power drugs can hold over us? These are but a few of the issues explored in this far-ranging series.

Educating people about the dangers of drugs can go a long way towards minimizing the desperate consequences of substance abuse for individuals and society as a whole. Luckily, human beings have the resources to solve even the most serious problems that beset them, once they make the commitment to do so. As one keen and sensitive observer, Dr. Lewis Thomas, has said,

> There is nothing at all absurd about the human condition. We matter. It seems to me a good guess, hazarded by a good many people who have thought about it, that we may be engaged in the formation of something like a mind for the life of this planet. If this is so, we are still at the most primitive stage, still fumbling with language and thinking, but infinitely capacitated for the future. Looked at this way, it is remarkable that we've come as far as we have in so short a period, really no time at all as geologists measure time. We are the newest, youngest, and the brightest thing around.

# MENTAL DISTURBANCES

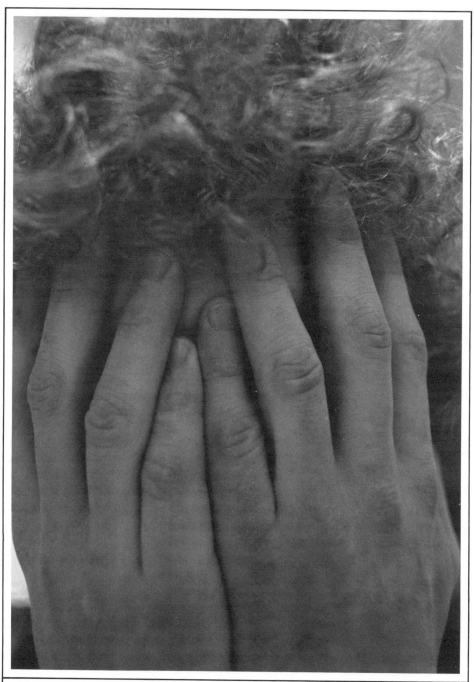

Mental illness afflicts some 35 million Americans from all walks of life. Recognizing the warning signs of these conditions and then seeking help are essential steps toward recovery.

# AUTHOR'S PREFACE

Is there a woman, man, or teenager who has not asked at some point, "Am I going crazy?"

Most people go through a period when they wonder if they might not be losing their grip on reality. It may be a time of sunken spirits, wild elation, deep anxiety, or a sudden surge of unexplained fear. Or it might be some seemingly silly ritualistic habit, a vague feeling someone is out to get them, or even persistent, unexplained aches and pains. These are all perfectly normal experiences in life.

But it is perfectly true that each of these emotional and physical states can be a symptom of mental disturbance. Any number of medical ailments can be diagnosed by a physical examination, laboratory tests, or X rays. However, the state of the human mind is a continuum, and psychiatrists and psychologists have yet to devise a precise way of telling when "normal" fades into "abnormal." As Solomon H. Snyder, M.D., of the Johns Hopkins University School of Medicine remarks in his book, *The Troubled Mind: A Guide to Release from Distress*, "The border between madness and sanity is a fuzzy one." And so it is not surprising that people may wonder occasionally about the state of their own mental health.

The effects of many illicit drugs mimic the terrifying mental distortions and symptoms of certain psychiatric illnesses. Cocaine can trigger hallucinations, anxiety, and paranoia. Chronic amphetamine use may result in a schizophrenialike illness. LSD (lysergic acid diethylamide) can produce severe anxiety, terrifying delusions, and profound fears of going insane. Phencyclidine (PCP or "angel dust") is notorious for causing bizarre and violent behavior, hallucinations, and muscle rigidity. In fact, in areas where PCP is now the hard drug of choice, it is found in the urine of 70% of the people admitted to psychiatric emergency units.

Of course, the existence of mental illnesses far predates the current epidemic of drug abuse. Psychiatric disorders have fascinated and terrified humans throughout history. Some mentally ill people have been raised to the status of prophets; many more have been cursed and condemned as possessed by evil spirits. Although our understanding of mental disturbances has deepened tremendously over the past century, many mysteries remain about their causes; often the diseases are resistant to cure, or treatment fails for reasons unknown. In addition, there remain many myths, superstitions, and prejudices that haunt the victims of these disorders and inhibit their recovery.

Psychiatrists and psychologists take their responsibility for diagnosing and treating mental illness quite seriously. Mental disorders are illnesses as sure as infections, allergies, asthma, heart disease, and cancer. Yet many people do not view them that way — not the public at large nor the patient whose mind has slipped from the path we call normal. A diagnosis of mental illness can be devastating to many people. In part, their attitude reflects a prevailing view within society — that one who suffers from a sickness of the mind is somehow less human than the person who suffers a sickness of the body.

At any given moment, millions of people within the United States alone are suffering from at least one mental disturbance. The aim of this volume is to acquaint people with some of the major psychiatric illnesses as well as some that particularly affect teenagers. It certainly is not intended as a diagnostic manual, and no one should attempt to diagnose themselves or anyone else based on what is contained here. Recognizing and treating mental disorders require considerable study and training. Because of society's unfortunate view of the mentally ill, carelessly to label another person as sick of mind — either as a joke or for some other reason — can have very damaging consequences.

Also beware of "medical students disease," sometimes called "medical writers syndrome." This is a curious phenomenon well known in medical schools. It is common for medical students and medical writers, early in their careers, suddenly to feel they have the disease they are studying no matter how bizarre the symptoms or how rare the ailment. (An eminent blood specialist once confessed to me that as a medical student he looked at his own white blood cells under the microscope and knew instantly he had leukemia. It turned out he was indeed ill—but with mononucleosis, not cancer.)

One thing you should not dismiss, however, is a friend who talks about suicide. Never ignore such talk, no matter how unbelievable it may be that someone you know would kill himself. Do not fall for that tragic myth that people who talk about suicide do not commit it. Many suicides do indicate their intentions beforehand. They may say so directly or hint at their intentions indirectly. They might make such remarks as "The world would be better off without me" or "I'd be better off dead."

If a friend gives any indication of suicide, offer a sympathetic ear and a willingness to talk about what is troubling him. Try to be reassuring, caring, and encouraging during any conversation. As painful for you as it may be, let the person keep talking. Do not change the subject or leave until your friend is finished. Talking often can relieve some of the pressure he is feeling. But avoid arguments and comments, such as "look how lucky you are," that might make your friend feel more depressed or guilty.

Empathy is wonderful, but it is not enough. Any suicide threat or hint at self-destruction should be treated seriously. Suggest that your friend call a suicide prevention center or crisis hotline or talk with a trusted adult — a parent, teacher, minister, or doctor. If the reaction is negative, then make the contact yourself to seek advice. Do not worry about betraying a friend's confidence and trust. You may well be saving a life, or at least putting a very unhappy life on the right path. Remember, people who talk about suicide are often suffering severe depression. They may feel overwhelmed by a sense of worthlessness and see no hope whatsoever that things will ever get better.

You may be the one that makes the difference.

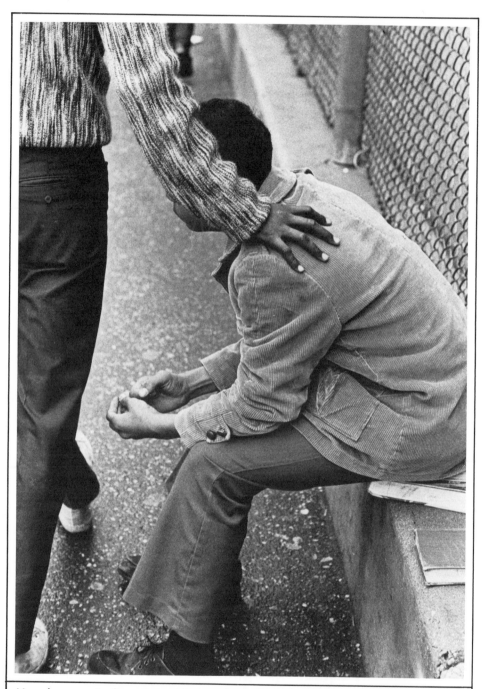

Hopelessness is the most ominous sign of severe depression, an illness that can lead to suicide if left untreated. Offering sympathy to a troubled friend can make the difference between life and death.

# CHAPTER 1

# DEPRESSION AND MANIA

To the outside world, James L. was a respected scientist in his mid-forties, much honored for his contributions to biomedical research. Yet the inner world of this brilliant man was in turmoil when he finally poured out to a psychiatrist his consuming fear that some degenerative disease was destroying his brain. He lacked the energy to work and could not sleep at night. His mind lost its creative edge, his ideas were uninspired and unimportant, and he saw no hope that he would ever again do worthwhile research. His thoughts dwelled on a friend who had hanged himself, and he confessed that on air flights he wished the plane would crash.

James L. was suffering from severe depression, the most common and the most life-threatening of the serious mental illnesses. Many people who commit suicide are suffering from depression at the time. Fortunately, depression is one of the more treatable mental disturbances. Drug treatments and psychotherapy helped restore James L.'s mental balance and free him from his fears and despair.

"I'm depressed" has become an American cliché, used to describe almost any mood that is not buoyant. But true depression is not simply "the blues" or the normal sadness of bereavement. It is a devastating illness that lasts for many

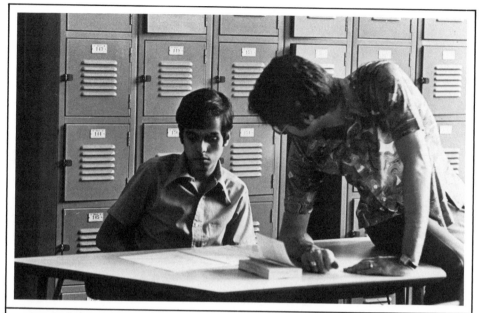

*A rehabilitation counselor works with a troubled adolescent. Although affective disorders usually afflict adults, younger people are also vulnerable to mild to severe depression.*

months if left untreated. Depression and a related problem called manic-depressive illness are known as "affective," or mood, disorders. Indeed, both are marked by major disturbances in mood. Depressives exhibit severe dejection; manics seem highly elated. A person who experiences only low moods suffers depression, or in the more formal psychiatric term, unipolar depression. Someone whose mood swings from soaring highs to deep lows, or who experiences only the highs of mania, is classified as suffering bipolar depression. Both are serious illnesses that can disrupt and destroy lives. A third affective disorder is called dysthymia, in which many symptoms of depression are present, but with less severity.

National statistics on mental illness are not very precise. But based on the Epidemiologic Catchment Area Program, the largest study ever made of mental disorders in the United States, the National Institute of Mental Health estimates that about 6% of Americans age 18 and over are suffering from an affective disorder at any given time. This includes .7% in the midst of mania, 3.1% suffering a major depressive episode, and 3.2% with dysthymia. According to this study, women are diagnosed with affective disorders about 1.4 times as often as men.

Although affective disorders usually afflict adults, they sometimes strike teenagers. In recent years, a number of researchers have concluded that younger children occasionally become severely depressed, even to the point of suicide.

## *"All My Dreams Have Died."*

People in the midst of depression often describe themselves as sad, discouraged, despondent, worried, or fearful. They are generally passive and dependent, and they often view themselves as worthless and living lives without pleasure. Many blame themselves for everything that goes wrong in their family and professional lives, even in the lives of total strangers. They consider their accomplishments as flukes or undeserved luck. Many feel their lack of ability or talent will eventually be discovered, and they will be exposed as the frauds they believe themselves to be. But the most ominous sign — the major symptom of severe and possibly life-threatening depression — is a lack of hope. As one patient said, explaining why he wished his life would end, "All my dreams have died."

Some depressed people initially see a physician because of one of the physical symptoms associated with the disorder. These include insomnia, early-morning awakenings, loss of energy, tiredness, poor appetite, constipation, agitation, irritability, loss of interest in sex, a slowing of thinking, an inability to focus attention, memory problems, reduced coordination, and a slowing of the body's response times. Sometimes the memory problems, particularly in the depressed elderly, are so profound that they are mistakenly diagnosed as having a dementia—a loss of mental capacity and emotional stability caused by damage to the brain. Dementia is not reversible; depression is.

Some severely depressed individuals suffer paranoid symptoms, hallucinations, and delusions. Their sense of guilt or evil is so overpowering that they feel the entire world hates them and seeks to harm them. Their hallucinations (hearing and seeing things that are not there) and delusions (beliefs that logic and reason prove are false) tend to focus on such things as punishment, disease, and death. In a typical delusion, they may feel they are so despicable that painful tortures and punishments will strike them. In their hallucinations they may hear what they believe is the voice of God condemning them for their evil.

The deeply depressed rarely have any hope or expectation that they will get better. Because of this, they may resist suggestions that they seek help and even reject it when it is offered. Some people suffer mild to moderate depression for much of their lives, some become depressed periodically, and some suffer one episode and never another. It is a hallmark of depression that people who slide to its depths almost always get better eventually, or at least experience periodic remission, even without treatment.

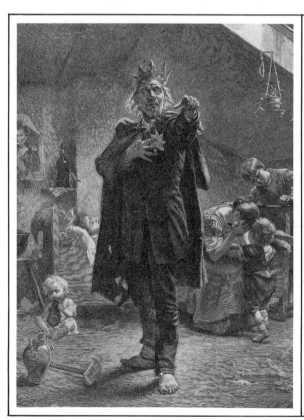

A 19th-century engraving entitled Delusions of Grandeur. *In severe cases of mania, hallucinations may occur in which the manic feels himself to be the source of great power or the carrier of a message from God.*

## Depression Flipped on End

To many, mania appears to be depression flipped on end. The typical manic — in contrast to the dour depressive — is euphoric, hyperactive, and overflowing with ideas. Everyone is the manic's friend; jokes and good times abound. Most manics talk nearly incessantly, pouring out an almost endless stream of understandable but disjointed ideas. During a mild attack, manics may produce amazing amounts of work and creative ideas. They can go for days with little or no sleep and without feeling tired or showing fatigue.

Appealing as this may sound, mania can be as hellish as depression. Manics display notoriously poor judgment and frequently act impulsively to their own detriment. Expensive shopping sprees, ruinous investment and business decisions, unwise career changes, and disastrous sexual exploits are common during mania. As an attack deepens, the manic may become irritable, disorganized, and incoherent. Delusions and hallucinations may occur in which the manic is the source of great power, influence, creativity, or a message from God.

Few bipolar depressives suffer only mania. Most are manic-depressives who swing between mania and depression, often with normal periods in between. Some suffer mania and depression simultaneously. As a rule, bipolar depression occurs at an earlier age than the unipolar type. Most bipolar depressives have their first episode in their late twenties. Unipolars are more likely to suffer their first depression after age 37.

## Depression and Suicide

Suicide is the 10th leading cause of death in the United States. But it ranks third — behind accidents and homicides — as the leading killer of teenagers and young adults. Boys are six times more likely to commit suicide than girls. Exactly why people kill themselves remains unknown, as does the reason why the suicide rate has tripled among those aged 15–24 since the mid-1950s.

Nonetheless, a significant number of people who kill themselves show signs of a psychiatric disorder before their deaths. The most frequent problem is bipolar or unipolar depression. Studies suggest that 50–70% of people who commit suicide are depressed. About 15% of severely depressed individuals eventually kill themselves. Surprisingly, the danger is not highest when depression is greatest but when the illness is improving. Some psychiatrists have suggested this is because the interest in living has not yet returned but the energy to plan and commit suicide has. The great hope is that treating severe depression will cut this tragic toll of self-destruction.

Manic-depressives are more likely to kill themselves than people who only get depressed. The reason for this difference remains unknown. Research suggests that people who commit suicide — whether depressed or not — tend to be more impulsive in their behavior, and bipolars are more impulsive than unipolar depressives.

## Subtypes of Depression

Psychiatrists and clinical psychologists widely agree that depression is not a uniform illness but a term that covers at least several disorders. There is less agreement on how to classify these various subtypes of depression precisely. Nonetheless, some useful distinctions are made. As we shall see, they are important in selecting treatment.

First, there are primary and secondary depressions. A depression is called primary when it occurs in someone who has never suffered another form of mental disturbance. But depression is also a frequent companion illness in hysteria, panic attacks, and alcoholism and may occur along with almost every psychiatric disorder. When depression occurs in someone with another mental illness, it is called secondary. People with secondary depression are less likely to commit suicide than those with primary depression.

Another useful distinction is between endogenous and exogenous depression. Endogenous (inner) depression appears to rise from within individuals and may occur without any stressful event in their lives. (An intriguing finding is that many of the sufferers of endogenous depression are struck by the disease after scoring a notable success — some career achievement, for example.) Exogenous (outer) depression appears triggered specifically by life's stresses. Sometimes endogenous is called "psychotic" depression and exogenous is

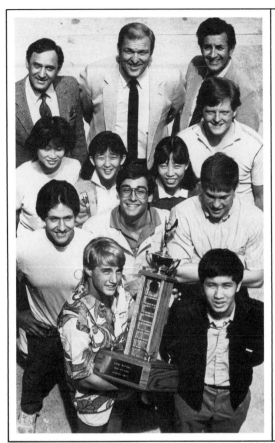

*Award-winning high school athletes and their coaches proudly display a trophy. Ironically, many people who suffer from depression are struck by the disease after scoring a notable success.*

referred to as "neurotic" depression. Exogenous depression is regarded as the milder of the two; its victims do not have as distorted an emotional outlook, their sleep is not disrupted, they experience fewer appetite and sexual problems, they do not suffer delusions or hallucinations, and they are less likely to kill themselves.

## What Causes Depression?

An argument raged for decades as to whether depression is a biological or psychological illness; whether it is caused by some biological defect in the body or grows out of events experienced in childhood. The turn-of-the-century German psychiatrist Emil Kraepelin believed depression and manic-depressive illness were "innate" — that is, biological — and occurred without social or psychological influence. Sigmund

Freud, who developed psychoanalysis to treat mental disorders, initially accepted this view. But he finally sided with Karl Abraham, who argued depression was a psychological illness that developed in people with an excessive need for nurturing, approval, and emotional support.

Today there is growing acceptance that depression and manic-depressive illness are complex disorders that involve biological, psychological, and social factors. No specific biological cause or defect has been linked to depression — no bacteria or virus, no abnormal hormone, enzyme, or other body chemical. But strong evidence indicates that the disorder is somehow related to changes in certain chemicals in the brain called neurotransmitters, which help pass messages from one nerve cell to another. These changes may result from some inherited genetic defect, or they may occur for other reasons. The two neurotransmitters most often implicated are serotonin and norepinephrine.

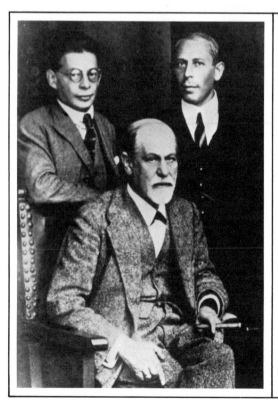

*Sigmund Freud, the father of psychoanalysis (foreground), with colleagues Otto Rank (left) and Karl Abraham. Freud and Abraham believed that depression is primarily a psychological rather than a biological disorder.*

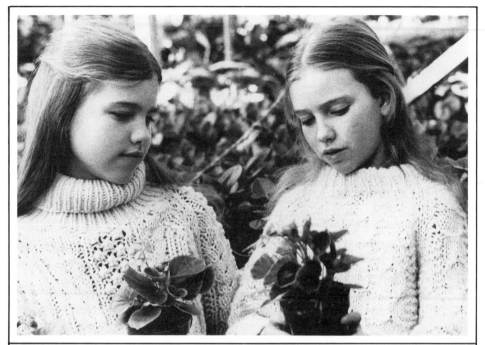

*Studies of identical twins, whose genetic makeup is exactly the same, indicate that although the disease of depression is not hereditary, a predisposition to suffer some of its symptoms is.*

Primary affective disorders tend to run in families. If your mother, father, sister, or brother has suffered depression or manic depression, your risk is greater than someone whose close relatives have not. The evidence that at least some depression is hereditary comes largely from studies of identical twins, whose genetic makeup is exactly the same, and fraternal twins, who, like nontwin siblings, share some but not all the same genes. If a disease were strictly genetic, you would expect that both identical twins would get the disease if one did, which would indicate a concordance rate of 100%. Identical-twin studies show a concordance rate of about 70% for manic depression and 40% for unipolar depression. Thus, what is inherited is not the disease itself but a tendency to it. Moreover, heredity plays a stronger role in bipolar depression than in unipolar. In 1987, researchers from three American universities reported evidence that a particular gene played a role in triggering manic depression.

That some people never suffer an affective disorder even though their identical twin does is evidence that environmental factors in life must play some role, as well. Again, these have not been precisely defined. But people who suffer depression tend to share two things: They have a greater need for nurturing and approval, and they harbor deep anger with themselves. Manic-depressives appear to be very dependent people who feel inferior and pour great effort into winning the acceptance of others. Moreover, the psychiatrist Aaron T. Beck, University Professor of Psychiatry at the University of Pennsylvania, has outlined a pattern of distorted thinking common to depressives. Among other traits, they view the world in black-and-white terms; they dwell excessively on negative events; and they anticipate that bad things will happen to them rather than good. In addition, Beck has developed a form of cognitive therapy called cognitive behavior therapy for victims of depression.

Thus, a combination of evidence supports the idea that depression involves both nature and nurture.

## Getting Help

Fortunately, depression responds well to treatment. Treating depression always requires psychotherapy to reassure the patient he or she will get better. Simply put, talking helps. A number of different types of psychotherapies are used, and studies find most are about equally effective. Psychotherapy may be all that is needed in the case of someone with mild and sometimes moderate depression. But talk alone is not effective for people with severe depression or mania. In such cases, psychotherapy is combined with drugs and sometimes electroconvulsive therapy (ECT), which is best known as shock treatment.

Drugs in use in the 1980s can shorten depressive episodes, ease the intensity of symptoms, and may even prevent new episodes. Two classes of medications are used: the tricyclic antidepressants and the monoamine oxidase (MAO) inhibitors. Both apparently act by increasing the supplies of the neurotransmitters norepinephrine and serotonin in the brain. Unfortunately, it takes two to four weeks before these drugs take full effect and lift the numbing symptoms of depression.

Undesirable side effects of tricyclic antidepressants, such as drowsiness, dry mouth, blurry vision, difficulty in urinating, and tremor, are usually not serious, although occasionally potentially serious abnormal heartbeats occur. The MAO inhibitors pose a more serious threat and are used much less frequently than tricyclics. MAO destroys not only norepinephrine but also tyramine, a chemical found in certain wines, cheeses, and other foods. High levels of tyramine increase blood pressure. Because MAO inhibitors prevent tyramine's destruction, the drugs can indirectly cause high blood pressure, severe enough in rare instances to cause sudden death.

For many years, doctors treated mania with large doses of barbiturates or tranquilizers, relying on their sedative effects to slow manics down. Chlorpromazine, a major tranquilizer, is still used in treating some cases of mania. But the most common treatment is lithium, a metallic element whose

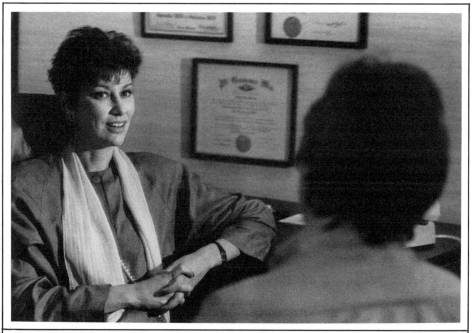

*A psychologist and her patient. Talking therapy is effective in the treatment of mild and sometimes moderate depression. In severe cases, however, psychotherapy is usually combined with drugs.*

healing powers were discovered in the late 1940s by John Cade, M.D., an Australian psychiatrist. Lithium has proved to be quite effective; many manic-depressives who consistently use prescribed doses of the drug not only do not suffer manic episodes but also avoid the severe depression that is part of their disorder. In addition, it seems that long-term lithium use reduces what was once a high rate of suicide among the victims of the disease. A recent survey found only 4 suicides among more than 9,000 manic-depressives who have been maintained on lithium for between 5 and 10 years.

Physicians, however, have wondered how this single drug could tame both the powerful highs and deep lows of bipolar depression. In 1986, Solomon H. Snyder and several colleagues at the Johns Hopkins University School of Medicine discovered a partial answer. Unlike tranquilizers and antidepressants that work on the surface of nerve cells, lithium works inside the cell. There it inhibits one of the "second messenger" systems involved in the complex process by which nerves communicate with one another. With that entire system dampened, so are the wild mood swings of the manic-depressive.

Lithium is a potentially toxic agent whose levels in the blood must be checked regularly. Even at therapeutic doses, lithium can cause a slight trembling of the hands, and long-term use may harm the kidneys and thyroid. At higher levels, it can cause disorientation, seizures, and death.

ECT is not a cure, but it may be the most effective treatment for depression. In ECT, patients are given an anesthetic and a muscle relaxant. Brief pulses of electricity are then passed through the brain from one electrode placed on the head to another, creating a seizure that lasts about a minute. Treatment generally consists of from six to a dozen ECT sessions, each two or three days apart. How ECT works remains a mystery. But it is as good as drugs at lifting depression, often works faster, and is probably no more dangerous. ECT is not very effective in treating mania.

Patients emerging from ECT typically have a headache, some confusion, and muscle fatigue. More important, they usually suffer a temporary loss of recent memory. This amnesia problem can be reduced by setting the electrodes on only one side of the head, a technique called unilateral ECT, rather than on opposite sides. Because of memory loss and the public's unfavorable perception of ECT, the therapy is used far less frequently than medications. It is generally reserved for victims of depression who do not respond to drugs, who are suicidal, or who are too mentally ill to be treated outside a hospital.

Many people envision ECT as an inhuman torture inflicted on unwilling mental patients — an image popularized by Sylvia Plath's novel *The Bell Jar* and the motion picture made from the Ken Kesey novel *One Flew Over the Cuckoo's Nest*. ECT once did cause frequent spinal compressions, bone fractures, and other injuries before anesthetics and muscle relaxants came into use. But the dangers have lessened as the therapy has become more sophisticated — an achievement that has not been reflected in a better public perception.

Whether a person is suffering endogenous or exogenous depression makes a difference in selecting treatment. Endogenous depressives do much better with drugs and ECT than exogenous depressives, whereas those with exogenous depression fare better with psychotherapy than do endogenous depressives.

Certainly there is no one perfect treatment for sufferers of either depression or manic depression. Debates still continue as to whether these conditions are due more to psychological or physical factors, to what extent psychotherapy helps, and whether these illnesses can be controlled solely by drugs. In addition, the medicines that treat these disorders have negative side effects that can be unpleasant and sometimes dangerous. Nevertheless, the progress scientists have made regarding the identification and possible treatment of these two forms of depression have been astonishing and certainly point to the development of even more effective medications in the future.

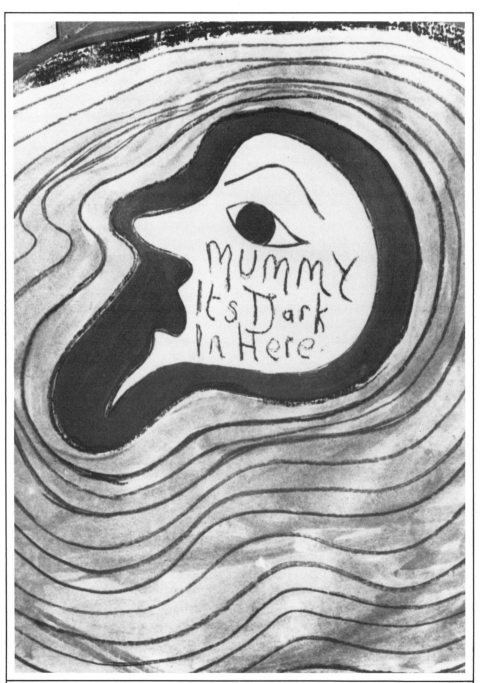

"Mummy it's dark in here," wrote the 25-year-old schizophrenic who did this drawing. Experts believe that schizophrenia is the most debilitating of all the mental illnesses.

# CHAPTER 2

# SCHIZOPHRENIA

**P**eople emerging from a Washington, D.C., subway station one morning found a bearded young man with long blond hair, flowing robes, and sandals proclaiming himself to be Jesus Christ. He shouted; he grimaced; he waved his arms as if summoning powerful demons. A few people paused to stare. Most hurried away, uncomfortable, and perhaps a little frightened by this dramatic encounter with the madness we call schizophrenia.

Most people think of the schizophrenic when they talk of someone being crazy. Victims of this mental disorder speak in a vague, disconnected way, making no logical connection between one statement and another. Their behavior is often so bizarre that people recoil and flee from them. Yet despite their chaotic rhetoric and eccentric ways, some schizophrenics have attracted followers who have regarded them as prophets or great leaders.

Schizophrenia is clearly the most disabling of all mental illnesses, a horrifying plight for its victims and those who love them. The schizophrenic feels as if his very "self" is disintegrating. "Many times I have felt that I was fighting my way up a dirt hill, and as I walked the ground crumbled beneath me, and I could make no movement," one young woman wrote. Mentally cut off from reality, schizophrenics withdraw emotionally and often physically from family, friends, and the world around them.

Delusions, hallucinations, and strange behavior are hallmarks of schizophrenia. Typically, the delusions involve persecution and control. Schizophrenics often fear they are the victims of conspiracies and that people — from the FBI, some other government agency, or even another planet — are spying on them. They may worry that outside forces are reading their minds and controlling their thoughts and actions. Some feel they have a message for the world — a way to international peace, a plan that will "save the government." They may even come to believe they are a famous religious or political personage — Jesus Christ, the Virgin Mary, Napoleon Bonaparte, Julius Caesar, Cleopatra, the president of the United States.

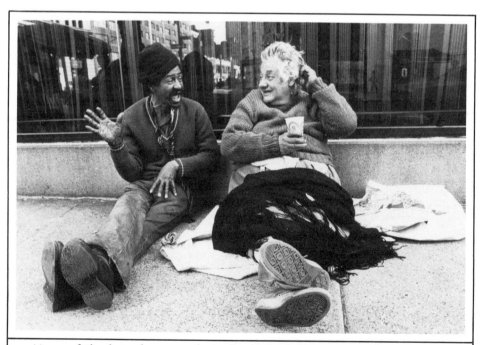

*Many of the homeless people in the United States are schizophrenic. Some argue that the greatest compassion would be to institutionalize these people so that they could receive medication and physical care.*

Hearing voices is the most common hallucination among schizophrenics. The voices may be of someone known or unknown to the schizophrenic. They may threaten or criticize or mock. They may command the person to do something he knows is wrong. Sometimes hearing voices follows a period when the person senses that his thoughts are being transmitted so that everyone knows what he is thinking.

Schizophrenics commonly suffer visual distortions: vague, terrifying forms, visions of dead relatives, bloody scenes of destruction, or fiery images from hell. A few victims experience olfactory (relating to the sense of smell) hallucinations, usually distasteful odors they sense are coming from their own bodies.

Although delusions and hallucinations are the most striking symptoms of schizophrenia, some victims never suffer either. Indeed, less dramatic but more persistent disturbances that blunt the emotions and intellectual capacities of schizophrenics appear to be at the core of the illness. The mind of the schizophrenic seems to shrink from the world outside. As the person retreats further, curiosity disappears, emotions, ideas, and the use of language diminish, and apathy and inertia prevail. Psychiatrists speak of the schizophrenic's "flattened" mood — emotional unresponsiveness, a lack of warmth and empathy, an ability to describe the most gruesome scene in a dry monotone. One psychiatrist tells how a patient recounted the gory death of his mother beneath the wheels of a car "without the faintest indication of strong emotion." Some schizophrenics develop what are called *autistic* symptoms — prolonged periods of silence and immobility and a progressive withdrawal from even those dearest to them.

Schizophrenia is usually chronic. Typically, it comes on gradually, so it is difficult to say just when it began, and it lasts to one degree or another for life. Most schizophrenics are hospitalized at least once — usually more frequently — for their illness. Some live out their lives in mental institutions. None escapes without serious disruption in their relations with their family and others; many never marry. Their illness prevents much success in education or career. Usually, when they can work, they hold menial jobs. A number of the homeless "street people" in American cities are schizophrenics. Yet, surprisingly, the rate of suicide is only slightly increased among people with this devastating mental disorder.

Schizophrenia exists among all races and cultures and in all countries. Researchers estimate that about 1% of the U.S. population becomes schizophrenic sometime during their life. The Epidemiologic Catchment Area study put the number suffering from the disorder at any one time at .9% of the adult population.

No one knows the cause of schizophrenia. The first recognizable symptoms generally appear in the late teens or early twenties; males tend to show signs a few years younger than females. Only rarely does the disease appear after age 45.

## What Is Schizophrenia?

Some experts believe that schizophrenia has always plagued the human race. Others argue that it is a disease that has developed in modern times. Emil Kraepelin first distinguished the disorder from other mental illnesses in the late 1800s. The term schizophrenia was coined in 1908 by the Swiss psychiatrist Eugen Bleuler. Literally, schizophrenia means "splitting of the mind." By this Bleuler meant an inappropriate splitting of the mind's functions — not a multiple or split personality of the sort portrayed in the motion pictures *The Three Faces of Eve* and *Sybil*. Actually, it is closer to the truth to say that the schizophrenic has no personality.

Although we speak of schizophrenia in the singular, most experts believe it is actually a series of disorders — different but related. Attempts to define the subtypes precisely have largely failed. Nonetheless, there is general agreement on three basic categories.

**Hebephrenic:** This term is derived from Hebe, the comical cupbearer to the gods in Greek mythology who always nipped at the wine as she made her rounds. Hebephrenics tend to behave in silly ways, but their grimaces, giggles, odd rhymes, and jokes are pathetic rather than funny. Delusions and hallucinations are not a major part of their symptoms. Yet their mental and emotional worlds are shattered. The onset of their illness is gradual, and its course is almost always unremitting. They often deteriorate into a chronic illness that plagues them for the rest of their life. Rarely do they experience significant remission.

**Catatonic:** The body behaviors of catatonics are dramatic, ranging from almost complete immobility to rapid, excited motion. They may adopt strange, statuesque positions and remain fixed for hours with expressions that suggest they have lost all touch with reality, or their movements may be jerky and machinelike, as if they were programmed robots. Their motions may be frenzied; they may run around, bang the wall or floor, and cry, scream, or sing loudly. Often catatonic schizophrenics alternate these behaviors. Some may not speak for months and even refuse to eat.

**Paranoid:** Paranoids are characterized by anxiety, anger, violent behavior, delusions of persecution or grandeur, and hallucinations. They tend to be more intelligent and alert than other types of schizophrenics, and their disease usually occurs a little later in life.

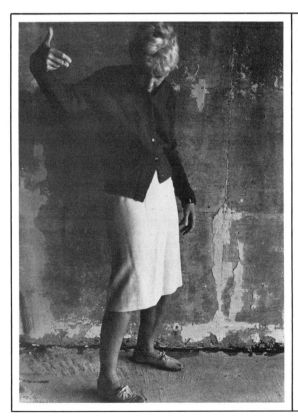

*A catatonic schizophrenic. Catatonics may strike strange, statuesque positions and remain frozen for hours.*

Precise as these categories sound, most schizophrenics exhibit overlapping symptoms. When a patient displays enough symptoms to fit more than one classification, the diagnosis is often undifferentiated schizophrenia.

## Nature Versus Nurture

The nature-versus-nurture argument — whether the disease is biologically inherited or caused by environmental factors — runs deep and heated in regard to schizophrenia. The disorder does tend to run in families. A child with one schizophrenic parent has about a 10% chance of developing the disorder; if both parents are schizophrenic, the chance is nearly 40%. But the tendency of the illness to occur in certain families could be explained by either biology or psychology. It could mean the disease is inherited, or it could mean certain families behave in such a way as to produce the illness in their children. It could involve both.

Nurture advocates believe that schizophrenia stems in large part from disturbed relations within the home, particularly problems in the mother-child relationship. Psychological writings have described so-called schizophrenogenic mothers, women whose coldness and rejection cause the disorder in their offspring. Indeed, studies do suggest that mothers of schizophrenics have unusual patterns of communication with their children. However, this could be an effect rather than the cause of schizophrenia; disturbed communications could result because the child destined to suffer schizophrenia acts abnormally from an early age, long before other symptoms appear. Today mothers are blamed less than in the past, which has helped reduce recriminations and anger within the families of schizophrenics, who often feel tremendous guilt that they are somehow personally to blame for the child's illness. Nonetheless, stresses within the family may play some role in schizophrenia.

Those who favor a biological cause of the disorder point to evidence suggesting that the brains of schizophrenics may be different from ordinary human brains and to studies of twins and adopted children that indicate a genetic factor.

In recent years, there have been major advances in the study of the living brain. Researchers have taken advantage

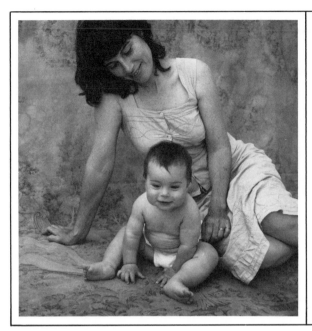

*A healthy mother and baby. Some experts believe that schizophrenia has its origins in profoundly disturbed relationships between young children and their mothers.*

of new techniques to look for specific brain abnormalities in schizophrenics. Some victims of this illness appear to have larger than normal cerebral ventricles (the cavities inside the brain). In others, a part of the brain called the cerebellar vermis seems smaller; or unusual physical or functional differences appear to exist between the right and left sides of the brain. Other studies suggest that the brains of some schizophrenics have abnormal patterns of blood flow, electrical activity, and glucose metabolism. At this point, however, no one knows what, if anything, these findings mean.

An intriguing recent discovery is that schizophrenics have an increased number of receptors for the neurotransmitter dopamine, whether or not they have been treated with antischizophrenic drugs. Receptors are molecules on the surfaces of cells to which drugs and body chemicals must attach in order to affect the cell. (Animal studies have suggested that drugs to treat schizophrenia increase the number of dopamine receptors in the brain.) Many experts believe that schizophrenia is the result of a hypersensitivity to dopamine in certain regions of the brain. There are several lines of evidence for this belief. Drugs used to treat the disorder apparently work by attaching to dopamine receptors, which prevents the dopamine from reaching them. Moreover, amphetamines increase the brain's production of dopamine and can trigger symptoms like those of schizophrenia. Nevertheless, the exact role of dopamine in the disorder remains unknown.

There is clear evidence that some people inherit a vulnerability to schizophrenia. Studies indicate that among identical twins, if one twin develops schizophrenia, the chance is about 50% that the other will, too. Among fraternal twins, that chance is between 10 and 15%. Several studies have also looked at children with at least one schizophrenic parent who were adopted and raised from an early age by people who did not suffer the mental illness. Consistently, more children with schizophrenic natural parents developed the disorder than did adopted children whose natural parents were not schizophrenic.

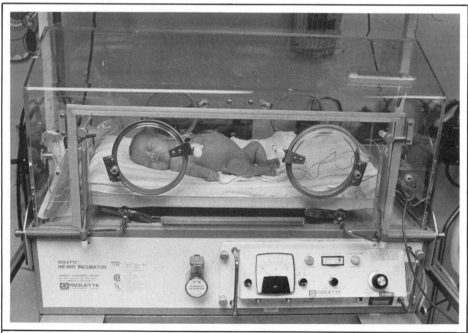

*A premature newborn in an incubator. Babies who are predisposed to schizophrenia are more likely to develop the disorder if they were afflicted with low birth weight.*

However, because there is not a total concordance, something other than genes must determine why an individual suffers from schizophrenia. It may be that no matter how much susceptibility they inherit, certain people do not become schizophrenic because they somehow avoid the psychological and other environmental events needed to push them over the line into madness.

What besides genes is involved? Although the answer is far from clear, in recent years researchers have begun to identify certain risk factors — situations or events that seem to increase the likelihood that someone genetically predisposed to schizophrenia will develop the disorder. These include problems at birth, such as an unusually low weight or an abnormal position during delivery; poor motor coordination or other neurological problems during infancy; poor emotional "bonding" between mother and infant; separation from parents at an early age; poor intellectual development, particularly problems in verbal abilities; difficulties in focusing attention; inability to get along with people; and confusion and hostility in the communications between parent and child.

## Drug Therapy

For decades there was little that could be done for schizophrenics except to hospitalize them, often for life, and try to calm them with barbiturates. Psychoanalysis and other types of psychotherapy failed to relieve their distorted thinking; neither drugs nor ECT could end their bizarre symptoms. Then, in the mid-1950s, a major advance in the treatment of schizophrenia emerged: a group of drugs known alternately as antipsychotics, major tranquilizers, or neuroleptics. The drugs were no cure, for most patients suffered relapses if they stopped taking them. But unlike barbiturates, these drugs actually lessened or controlled some of the disorder's severe symptoms — particularly hallucinations, delusions, and bizarre behavior. They proved far less effective with anxiety, agitation, social withdrawal, and the blunting of emotions. For some patients, the drugs failed to help at all.

Introduction of the antipsychotic drugs allowed the release of many schizophrenics from mental hospitals. Some returned to their families; others even went on to live rela-

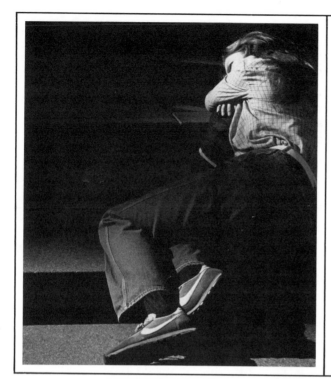

*Process schizophrenics, the most difficult to treat, are severely withdrawn in their behavior and are rarely, if ever, capable of having normal relationships with others.*

tively independent lives in the community. In spite of this, no group of mental patients spends more time in psychiatric hospitals than schizophrenics.

The drugs also cause serious side effects. Some people develop symptoms similar to those of Parkinson's disease — tremor, muscle rigidity, and movement problems. Others suffer akathisia, an inability to remain still that leads to frequent movement. Another serious problem is tardive dyskinesia, which causes excessive movement of the face muscles and tongue and grossly distorts the patient's appearance.

Drugs alone do not rehabilitate schizophrenics any more than psychotherapy can cure the illness. Yet together they can increase the ability of schizophrenics to function in society and improve their quality of life. Drugs control symptoms; psychotherapy and other support techniques build up what emotional strength the patient has. Unfortunately, such efforts are costly and not available to most schizophrenics, whose financial resources are usually meager.

About two-thirds of schizophrenics released from mental hospitals go to live with their family, most often their parents. The return of a schizophrenic can cause extreme emotional and financial problems within a household. There is always the social stigma of having someone mentally ill in the family as well as the problem of living day to day with someone whose behavior is, at best, abnormal. The patience and strength of even the most caring, loving parent can quickly deteriorate. Treating the schizophrenic often means providing understanding, support, encouragement, and guidance to the family, as well.

American psychiatrists refer to schizophrenics who make some recovery as "reactive" and those who do poorly as "process." Although it is difficult to determine immediately whether a schizophrenic is reactive or process, there are some general characteristics to consider in making a diagnosis. Reactive schizophrenia generally begins abruptly; process schizophrenia comes on gradually. Reactive schizophrenics tend to have exhibited normal behavior and formed normal relationships before their illness, and they are more likely to suffer vivid hallucinations and delusions. Moreover, schizophrenia does not tend to run in their families, although there is often an increased incidence of affective illnesses. Process schizophrenics, on the other hand, seem to always have been withdrawn in their behavior and never capable of normal relationships with others. There is also a high incidence of schizophrenia in their families.

The prognosis for schizophrenics is often unpredictable. Yet evidence is emerging in the United States and Europe that the outlook is not as bleak as believed only a few years ago. For example, when researchers followed up 118 schizophrenics released from a Vermont mental hospital 20–25 years earlier, they found that nearly half showed considerable improvement after participating in a supportive psychotherapy program. They were not cured; they were not well. However, they had improved — much more so than many psychiatrists would have expected.

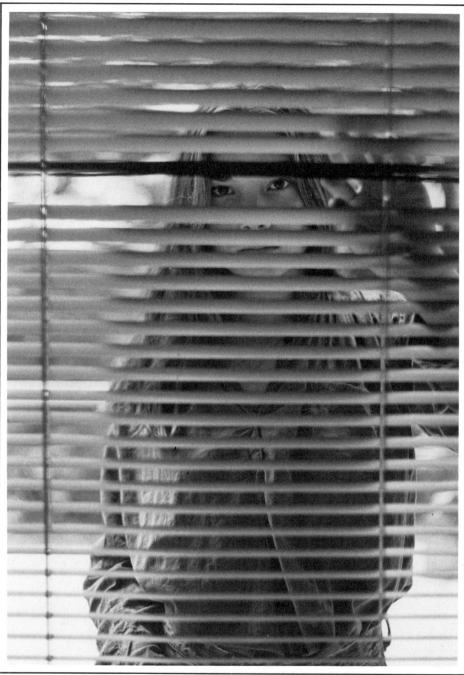

*Severe agoraphobia literally leaves its victims housebound. It is one of a cluster of mental disturbances known as anxiety disorders, the most common emotional problems in the United States.*

# CHAPTER 3

# ANXIETY, PANIC ATTACKS, AND AGORAPHOBIA

$S$heila T. suffered her first panic attack at the age of 17. She was at a shopping mall when suddenly, unexpectedly, she was seized by a terrifying sense of panic that sent her heart racing, set her body trembling, and left her gasping for breath. Sheila thought she was about to die.

The attack passed quickly but left her shaken and fearful. Another struck a few weeks later as she rode a bus, then another as she walked along a street, and yet another aboard a subway. Sheila began avoiding the kinds of places where her attacks had struck. She began to fear she was losing her mind and that total strangers would have her committed to an insane asylum. Finally, Sheila retreated to her home and simply stayed there, afraid, in time, even to answer the door. She did not go out again for four years. Sheila had developed severe agoraphobia — a fearful avoidance of particular places that literally leaves some people housebound.

Panic attacks and agoraphobia are part of a cluster of mental disturbances called anxiety disorders. Others within this category are generalized anxiety, social and simple phobias (Chapter 4) and obsessive-compulsive disorder (Chapter 5). Anxiety disorders are the most common mental problems in the United States. The Epidemiologic Catchment Area Program data indicated that 8.3% of American adults suffer from some anxiety — the distress and uneasiness that accompanies an apprehension of danger or misfortune. Anxiety that lasts hours or sometimes days is a normal part of life. But when the anxiety is severe and lasts more than a month, it is called generalized anxiety disorder, which may afflict as much as 4.5% of the nation's adults at any time.

## *Generalized Anxiety Disorder*

Generalized anxiety disorder, or GAD, is diagnosed when a person has suffered symptoms from three or four of the following categories for a month or more:

1. Motor tension, including shakiness, jumpiness, trembling, tension, muscle aches, inability to relax, eyelid twitch, and restlessness.
2. Autonomic hyperactivity, including sweating, racing heart, cold and clammy hands, dry mouth, dizziness, upset stomach, frequent urination, lump in the throat, and high pulse rate.
3. Apprehensive expectations, including worry, fear, and thoughts about and anticipation of misfortune to oneself or others.
4. Vigilance and scanning: excessive attentiveness that actually results in distraction, difficulty in concentrating, insomnia, feeling "on edge," irritability, and impatience.

Because GAD's symptoms mimic a number of physical disorders, it is important to first rule out such things as an overactive thyroid, low blood sugar, an adrenal-gland tumor called a pheochromocytoma, drug intoxication, excessive caffeine use, withdrawal from certain medications, and depression before saying someone has this mental disturbance.

GAD is among the more common reasons people visit physicians. Although this disturbance almost always goes away eventually, with or without treatment, while it lasts it can seriously disrupt lives, relationships, and work. The goal in treating GAD is to ease the symptoms so that the person can function normally and to help the patient cope with the stresses underlying the anxiety. Contrary to the popular notion that tranquilizers *cure* GAD, these drugs at best mitigate symptoms. They do not affect the underlying psychological cause. Drugs may play a useful role in GAD, but they are only part of a wider therapy program.

Treatment requires reassuring patients, identifying the stresses behind their anxiety, and teaching them to cope better with those stresses that cannot be eliminated. Psychotherapy may be used both to give a patient crucial emotional support and to determine the possible causes of the anxiety. Behavior techniques such as meditation, deep relaxation, and biofeedback can help relieve the adverse effects of stress. So can vigorous exercise, including jogging, aerobic dancing, or lap swimming. Although these approaches are sometimes effective by themselves, more often they are used in combination with drugs.

Minor tranquilizers called benzodiazepines became the drugs of choice for GAD in the 1960s, and one trade name became famous — Valium. Although generally safe and effective, the benzodiazepines also produce some unwanted and sometimes serious side effects. For example, they can cause coordination and memory problems and sedation, which can be a safety hazard on the job and while driving. They also are potentially addictive and can cause painful withdrawal

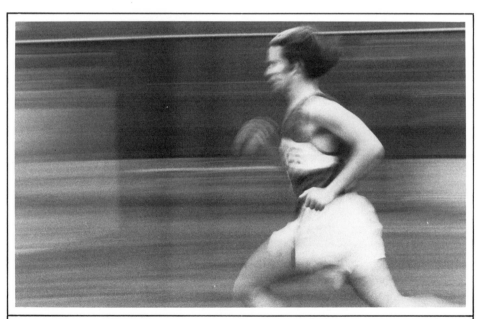

*A runner in full stride. Vigorous exercise—including jogging, aerobic dancing, and lap swimming—and certain behavior techniques such as meditation, can help relieve the adverse effects of stress.*

symptoms. There is, however, a new type of tranquilizer on the market. Called buspirone, this drug appears as effective as the benzodiazepines, but with fewer side effects, particularly those of sedation and dependence.

## Panic Attacks

Although many people who experience panic attacks also suffer generalized anxiety disorder, most experts no longer regard panic attacks — and the agoraphobia that sometimes results — as simply a form of GAD, but as a distinct disorder that is fundamentally different in both its nature and cause.

Debilitating panic attacks do in fact occur without another mental disturbance. When this happens, then the diagnosis of anxiety neurosis or panic disorder is made. Although Sigmund Freud coined the term "anxiety neurosis" in 1895, several European physicians had described the problem as early as the mid-1700s.

Panic is a normal human reaction that serves a vital function in that it creates a sudden burst of energy that can send a person fleeing safely from a life-threatening situation. But when this process occurs at inappropriate times — when there is no danger or any reason to suspect some harm or misfortune — it is a sign of abnormality.

Panic attacks almost always strike suddenly. They can occur at any time or place — in a crowded elevator or in bed. Without warning, a person feels foreboding, even terror. Fears of insanity or of a serious, perhaps fatal illness flash through the mind. Often there is a feeling that somehow the body itself has changed or become distorted. Someone in the midst of a "false alarm" panic suffers the same physical reactions as if he or she had suddenly encountered a coiled rattlesnake.

The heart races, breathing speeds up and becomes labored, and blurred vision, chest pain, dizziness, and even fainting, trembling, and sweating are common. The immediate physical responses generally last less than 30 seconds. But the experience can leave a person physically shaken and mentally drained for much longer. Often people with panic disorder suffer the symptoms of an attack in much milder form between full-blown attacks. When such people see a physician, their symptoms may be mistakenly diagnosed as heart ailments or gastrointestinal problems, such as an "irritable colon."

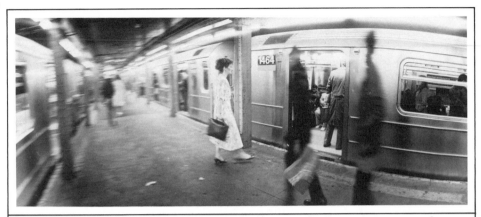

*A young woman on a New York City subway platform. Panic attacks can occur at any time or place. They usually strike suddenly, causing rapid breathing, chest pains, dizziness, and even fainting.*

Most people who suffer from panic disorder experience their first attack in their middle teens or twenties. The first attack rarely begins after age 35. Sometimes panic disorder comes "out of the blue," but most people, once diagnosed, remember experiencing such things as nervousness, tension, and dizzy spells for months or years before their initial attack. Secondary depression is a common complication of panic disorders, but suicides are rare. Indeed, most people who suffer panic attacks continue to function and live productive lives. Nonetheless, many also develop agoraphobia, which may run from mild to incapacitating.

### Agoraphobia

Agoraphobia once was thought to occur spontaneously. But psychiatrists and psychologists have come to realize that it is usually preceded by panic attacks. As a result, agoraphobia is now widely viewed as a consequence or complication of panic disorder. Actually, agoraphobia generally involves several phobias. In one sense, it is the fear of fear. That is, people with agoraphobia come to fear going to places where they have suffered panic attacks for fear they will suffer another attack there. For some, the disorder only slightly disrupts their lives. But at its most severe, agoraphobia can be as crippling as schizophrenia and extremely difficult to treat. Sheila T. lost her job, her marriage fell apart, and her relations with her close family suffered terribly. Even after a year of treatment she was able to return to work only sporadically.

The term agoraphobia was coined in 1871. *Agora* comes from the Greek word meaning "place of assembly" or "marketplace"; *phobia*, from the ancient Greek god Phobos, who inspired fear in all who looked at him. Literally, the term originally meant "fear of open places." But its victims may fear closed or open places — elevators, crowded rooms, cars, planes, bridges, tunnels, stores, and enclosed malls, as well as parks, streets, woods, or fields.

Among diagnosed agoraphobics, women outnumber men four to one. However, some researchers contend that such an unequal distribution between the sexes is not that significant. They believe that there are more diagnosed female agoraphobics than men simply because women are more likely to seek help than men. According to these researchers,

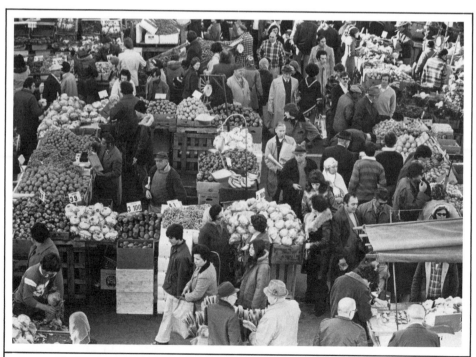

*Agoraphobia, the pathological fear of open spaces, is now considered a consequence or complication of panic disorder. The term comes from the Greek word* agora, *which means "place of assembly" or "marketplace."*

because it is less acceptable for men than for women to seek help, many male agoraphobics remain undiagnosed; they instead force themselves to go out and battle their intense anxiety with alcohol.

## What Causes Panic Disorder?

The cause of panic attacks remains uncertain, as does the reason why some people respond with agoraphobia and others do not. However, research indicates that both biology and psychology play a role in both problems.

Freud believed that most agoraphobics, particularly women, were people who were subconsciously avoiding impulses toward sexual abandon. This view long dominated the thinking of many American psychiatrists and influenced many popular articles written on the disorder. However, most psychologists abandoned Freud's theory early on and instead believed that agoraphobia could be learned behavior. The American psychologist John Watson suggested that a frightening experience in a certain place would be enough for a person to develop a subconscious fear of that place. In the 1980s, some psychologists believe that panic attacks develop when people, for whatever reason, misinterpret the potential danger of some unpleasant or unexpected body change — dizziness, a sudden increase in pulse rate, or an unusual heartbeat or two, for instance.

Both panic attacks and agoraphobia run in families. Perhaps 30–40% of agoraphobics have close relatives who have suffered anxiety disorders. Studies of twins indicate that both identical twins are more likely to suffer agoraphobia than both fraternal twins, suggesting that genes play some role. Indeed, it is now widely accepted that people inherit a predisposition to panic attacks, but psychological, social, and perhaps physical factors are needed to trigger the attacks in those individuals who are vulnerable.

Many people who suffer panic disorders report major stressful events in their lives six months or a year before the attacks begin. These include such things as the death of a loved one, job problems, a job change or loss, marriage, divorce, or a move to another city.

Perhaps as many as 50% of those who suffer panic attacks also have a condition called mitral-valve prolapse, in which

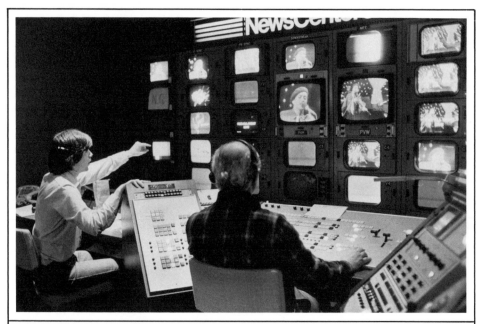

*Busy television technicians in front of their monitors. Most people handle routine job stress well, but undue pressure at work can sometimes result in serious panic disorders.*

a heart valve fails to close properly. This produces a so-called heart murmur and occasionally a rapid heart rate or abnormal beat. Another possible cause of panic attacks is caffeine. Thomas Uhde, M.D., and his colleagues at the National Institute of Mental Health found that caffeine equal to the amount contained in four or five cups of coffee triggered attacks in nearly half their panic-disorder patients. Moreover, some people who had never had a panic attack suffered one when given caffeine equal to that contained in seven or eight cups of coffee.

### Treating Panic Disorder

Rarely is intensive psychotherapy needed in treating panic attacks. But reassuring people that their problem does not threaten their life or mind and that it can be treated is important. Sometimes minor tranquilizers such as Valium are used for short periods. However, the tricyclic antidepressants have proved more effective for long-term treatment. Some doctors feel that these drugs work on underlying depression. However, most researchers believe there is some other effect involved, because the antidepressants are equally effective in treating a panic disorder in people who are not depressed. Propranolol is another drug sometimes used to treat panic attacks. It is one of a group of medications called beta-adrenergic blockers that are used to treat potentially life threatening abnormal heartbeats.

Drugs alone are rarely effective in the treatment of agoraphobia. They may suppress panic attacks, but they do not correct the psychological need to avoid certain places. Therefore, a combination of medication and psychological therapy is beginning to be used more frequently. Exposure therapy is the oldest and most commonly used nondrug treatment for agoraphobia. This involves "desensitizing" the person by reassuring him that there is no danger and gradually exposing the person to the place he fears. The exposure, at least initially, may be imaginary. The therapist persuades the person repeatedly to imagine doing something he fears — such as riding in an elevator — so he becomes more relaxed with the idea and later can go through the actual experience. Hypnosis is sometimes used to aid this imagery process.

In addition to his therapy designed to help depressives (see Chapter 1), Aaron T. Beck, a psychiatrist at the University of Pennsylvania, has developed a form of cognitive behavior therapy to treat agoraphobia. According to Beck, certain distorted ways of thinking lead people who suffer a panic attack to see it as a threat to their life or sanity. The goal of cognitive therapy is to enable patients to focus on and correct these responses. Psychologist David H. Barlow of the State University of New York, Albany, has developed another approach. In this therapy, agoraphobics simulate the actual symptoms they feel during a panic attack by imagining situations they fear or by vigorous exercise to get their hearts racing. Therapists then help them realize that their physical reactions are not really a threat to them. As Barlow has said, "These people are afraid of their own internal symptoms."

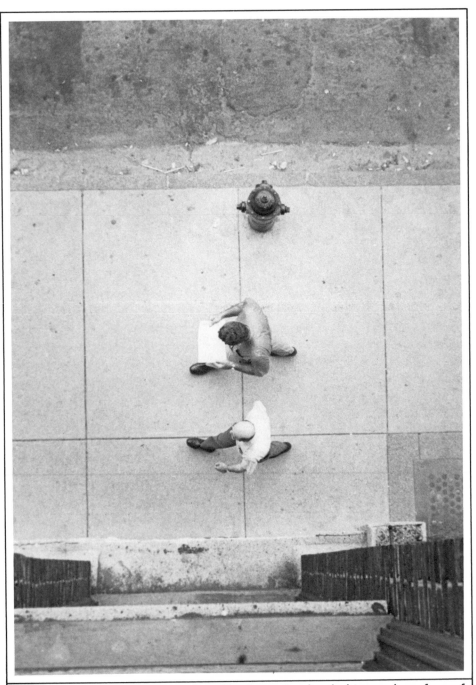

*Many otherwise healthy people suffer from simple phobias such as fear of heights. Chronic, powerful, and disruptive phobias, however, constitute a psychiatric disorder and should be treated.*

# CHAPTER 4

# SIMPLE AND SOCIAL PHOBIAS

Fred M. hates and fears the number 13. He avoids the 13th floor of buildings and driving or walking on streets or routes numbered 13. He hates to travel on Friday the 13th, particularly by airplane. He detests being in a room containing 13 people. (He counts.) Several times when he could not escape such gatherings, he began to feel tense and apprehensive. His chest tightened, he had mild breathing problems, and he felt his heart beating faster.

Fred M. suffers from a rare phobia — triskaidekaphobia, fear of the number 13.

Almost everyone has heard of phobias, but the term is often misused or misunderstood. A phobia is an anxiety reaction. It is an excessive, recurrent, and irrational fear that compels a person to avoid a specific object, activity, or situation.

Of course, fear is a normal part of life; phobias, however, are abnormal fears. Normal fear can be quite rational; phobias are unreasonable and disabling to one degree or another. In cases of mild phobia, sufferers may go for years or even through life without realizing their fear is abnormal. A sense of apprehension that strikes as they near a cliff or see a growling dog seems perfectly natural. However, when phobias are chronic and powerful enough to interfere with lives and careers — when people avoid things or situations in a disruptive way, such as never traveling on Friday the 13th — they are considered to have a phobic disorder that should be treated. A full-blown phobic disorder may develop over time, coming on so gradually a person has no idea when it began.

## Types of Phobias

Phobias are generally divided into three categories. We have already discussed agoraphobia, by far the most debilitating and difficult to treat, in Chapter 3. Less serious but still disruptive at times are the simple phobias and social phobias. A simple phobia is a morbid fear of an object, which can range from hair to rats to sunglasses. Victims of social phobias are haunted by the fear that they will be embarrassed in public by some specific act, such as speaking, writing, or eating.

Simple and social phobias often occur in otherwise normal and mentally healthy people. An abnormal fear may be their only mental quirk. But phobias also may accompany

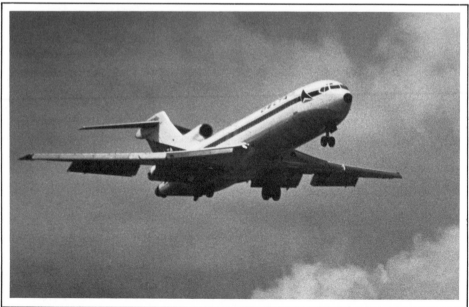

*Fear of flying is one of the most common of all phobias. Various therapies are proving successful in the treatment of such disorders.*

other psychiatric disorders. As we have seen, agoraphobia is usually a direct result of panic attacks. Simple and social phobias are found frequently among people with obsessive-compulsive behavior. (See Chapter 5.) Severe phobics may suffer secondary depression as a result of their illness.

The first known medical use of the term phobia was in ancient Rome some 2,000 years ago. However, the word phobia was not frequently used until the 19th century. An 1848 medical dictionary offered the word "syphiliphobia" and defined it as "a morbid dread of syphilis giving rise to fancied symptoms of the disease." Increasingly after that, a number of irrational and sometimes bizarre fears severe enough to attract the attention of physicians were given names derived from Latin or Greek ending with the root "phobia."

People can and do develop phobias to just about anything. Over the years, some very long lists have appeared. In his book *Nothing to Fear: Coping with Phobias* the medical writer Fraser Kent lists more than 300 specific fears. These run from A to Z — acarophobia (fear of mites, ticks, and small insects) to zoophobia (fear of animals) — and include cremnophobia (cliffs and precipices), esophobia (dawn), iatrophobia (doctors), pediophobia (dolls, mannequins, and dummies), and, of course, triskaidekaphobia. A list of names coined over the years to describe people's irrational fears — some common, some extraordinarily rare — is given in Appendix I.

The number of people who actually suffer from phobias, mild or severe, remains unknown. The Epidemiologic Catchment Area study estimated that at any given time 7% of the adult U.S. population is suffering from a phobia, including agoraphobia, severe enough to require treatment. Estimates in several other studies have put the proportion of Americans with some degree of phobia, from occasional symptoms to disabling attacks, at between 19% and 44%.

There are reasons for this wide range in estimates of incidence. First, there is no clear-cut boundary between an unusually strong fear and a mild phobia. Even the most astute authorities may disagree on when the line between normal and abnormal fear is crossed. Second, many people hide their phobias. They are embarrassed or ashamed by their fears —

even concerned friends or relatives may ridicule them or think they are crazy. Therefore they keep their phobias a secret, particularly some of the stranger ones.

A simple phobia is defined as a persistent, irrational fear that compels a person to avoid an object or situation. If a person avoids a place for fear he will not be able to escape when panic strikes, that is agoraphobia, not simple phobia. If the avoidance is because the individual fears being embarrassed or humiliated by some act in a social situation, that is a social phobia. Women suffer simple phobias more often than men; social phobias occur equally in both sexes.

Among the more common phobias are the fear of heights and — particularly in childhood — of animals. Others include fear of flying, blood, hypodermic needles, winds, storms, automobile driving, and loud noises. Some phobic objects can, indeed, cause harm. Cats scratch, dogs bite, and falling off a high cliff or building can be fatal. Even when an object does pose some potential threat, a phobic's fears are indiscriminate and totally out of proportion to the actual danger. The person with ophidiophobia makes no distinction between a deadly cobra and a harmless garter snake. Both evoke the same fearful response and avoidance.

Most people with simple phobias do not suffer any more or less anxiety in their lives than anyone else — until they are exposed to the specific object or situation they fear. Then their reaction may range from severe discomfort to the symptoms of a panic attack. Although the experience may be intense and cause the person to avoid the source of fear, people with simple phobias generally do not develop the anxieties found in social phobias and agoraphobia. Moreover, simple phobias are not always disabling. Some people can avoid their phobic object or situation without disrupting their lives. A thalassophobic living in Kansas, for example, is safe there from his fear of the sea or ocean.

A social phobia, as noted, involves a persistent, irrational fear that the person will embarrass or humiliate himself in public through some act. Some of the more common phobias include public speaking or eating, writing, or urinating in the presence of others. The American psychologist David Barlow has suggested that some male sexual problems are really social phobias stemming from men's concern about their ability to perform.

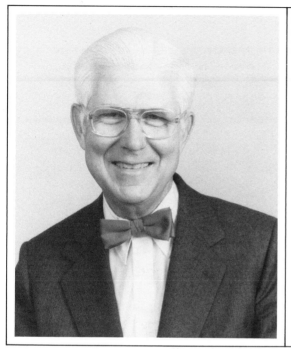

*Aaron T. Beck, M.D., University Professor of Psychiatry, University of Pennsylvania. Dr. Beck has developed a form of cognitive therapy that is proving successful in the treatment of some cases of agoraphobia and social phobias.*

Typically, social phobias cause only mild impairment and do not lead to complete avoidance of situations. Occasionally, avoidance is total, and social phobias do interfere with the enjoyment of life.

Simple phobias usually begin in childhood or early adolescence. In some people, they begin to improve after a few years and eventually disappear; in others, they remain throughout life. The earlier in life a simple phobia appears, the more likely it is that the person will lose it. Social phobias appear in adolescence or the early twenties. Rarely do they strike young children or after the third decade of life. Unfortunately, the chance of recovery without treatment is not as good for the social phobias. More often, they develop, stabilize for years, and then begin to lessen in intensity during middle age.

## What Causes Phobias?

The exact cause of simple and social phobias remains uncertain and is a matter of some contention. They seem related to early childhood fears that are transferred later in life to specific objects or situations. Unlike agoraphobia, simple and social phobias do not appear to run in families. If there are no genetic factors involved, then phobias must somehow emerge from a person's interaction with other people and the environment. Experts view simple and social phobias as psychological, not biological, disorders. Beyond that there are some sharp disagreements.

Freudians view phobias as expressions of repressed conflicts or impulses to forbidden acts. Locked away in the subconscious and unrecognized by the conscious mind, these repressed thoughts and urges manifest themselves as phobias. Thus, claustrophobia is seen as resulting from a child's fear of being abandoned and left in a small, enclosed space, usually nothing more dangerous than his bedroom. Fears of flying and driving are seen as repressed urges to kill or maim other people.

On the other hand, most psychologists and many non-Freudian psychiatrists view phobias as a form of learned or conditioned behavior. Some argue that a phobia grows out of a particularly frightening childhood experience that comes to be associated with a specific object or situation. Thus, the person comes to fear the thing associated with the early fright. Others suggest that at least some phobias serve as positive rewards for people and thus reinforce their behavior. A fear of flying, for example, may allow a person who does not want to be away from his family to remain close to home.

Drugs do not cure phobias. They may be used to relax people and reduce their fear during certain therapies or to relieve secondary depression. However, medications have not proved to be useful treatments for either simple or social phobias. Instead, most therapists believe a person must confront the feared object or situation to conquer the phobia. The idea is that phobias are learned fears that must be unlearned. By far the most popular approaches — the "exposure therapies"—are based on this learning theory.

## Exposure Therapies

•Systematic Desensitization: This is the most widely used exposure therapy. It involves gradually preparing the person to face his phobia. Over time, the person learns relaxation techniques and is exposed more and more to the feared object or situation. A person afraid of flying may first imagine driving to the airport. In the next session, he imagines the drive and entrance to the terminal building, and so on until he completes a mental flight. Eventually the phobic is expected to make an actual flight. Use of the imagination is intended to help the patient overcome the learned fear, but the key to defeating the phobia is confronting the actual object or situation in person.

•Modeling: This is a gentler approach. The patient watches other people, either in person or on videotape, functioning normally and without fear in a situation that fills him with terror. The therapist, for example, may sit petting a beagle while reassuring a person afraid of dogs.

•Flooding: Based on the notion that any fear has its limits, this technique involves intensely "flooding" the patient with the feared object or situation. There is no gradual buildup. A claustrophobic may be put in a closet or an acrophobic taken to the roof of a tall building — always with a therapist present. The idea is to force the phobic to experience his terror with maximum intensity. When he discovers that no harm has resulted from the experience, the fear begins to diminish, and the phobia relinquishes its hold.

Flooding, also called "implosion therapy," is not widely used, although some therapists report that it can be extremely effective in the treatment of simple phobias. Indeed, some therapists regard the technique as dangerous. They fear it could trigger other mental problems or even a heart attack.

Psychoanalysis continues to be used by some psychiatrists to help phobics gain insights into their subconscious thoughts and emotional conflicts. More recently, the cognitive behavior therapy that has shown promise in treating agoraphobia (see Chapter 3) is also being used with some success to treat social phobias, as well.

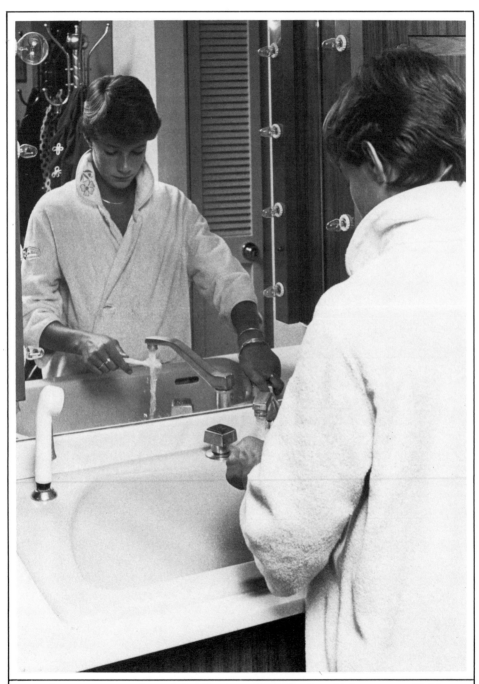

*Obsessive-compulsive behavior is a disorder in which uncontrollable thoughts often lead to ritualistic acts, such as repeated cleanliness routines. Such acts are senseless but relieve pent-up tensions.*

# CHAPTER 5

# OBSESSIVE-COMPULSIVE BEHAVIOR

Jamie A., an accomplished amateur chef, stopped cooking for his wife because he became overwhelmed by the fear that he would poison her. Myra F. lived in fear of dirt. The 12 year old began her cleansing rituals promptly at 6 A.M. each school morning. First, she spent half an hour shaking her clothing free of germs. Then she washed and rewashed her body, although somehow she never felt clean enough. By the time Myra sought medical help, she was spending six hours a day washing herself, sometimes until her skin bled.

Both Jamie and Myra suffered from obsessive-compulsive behavior, a psychiatric disorder in which uncontrollable thoughts often lead to ritualistic acts. Once thought the rarest of the major mental disturbances, obsessive-compulsive disorder now appears to be more common than anyone had ever suspected. Far from being essentially an affliction of late adolescence and young adulthood — as psychiatrists had long believed — increasing evidence indicates that a significant percentage of obsessive-compulsives are younger children like Myra F.

Obsessions are thoughts or impulses that are unwanted, persistent, distressing, senseless, even repugnant, and yet they defy attempts to ignore or suppress them. The key difference between an obsession and a delusion is that a person with an obsession makes a determined but unsuccessful effort to fight it. Compulsions are repetitive acts carried out as a result of obsession. They are unrealistically intended as a means of producing or preventing some future event. People with compulsions usually realize their ritualistic behaviors are senseless. (This is not always true of young children.) They get no pleasure from their activities, but they do get a temporary release from the tension within them. An obsessive-compulsive disorder exists if a person suffers chronic obsessions — with or without compulsions — that cause great mental distress and interfere with everyday life. Roughly 75% of people who are severely obsessed also experience compulsions.

Obsessive-compulsives were long regarded almost as oddities by psychiatrists. Such people are often secretive about their condition, and many prefer to live with their discomforting thoughts and acts rather than seek help. For years, therefore, it was estimated that only about .5% of the

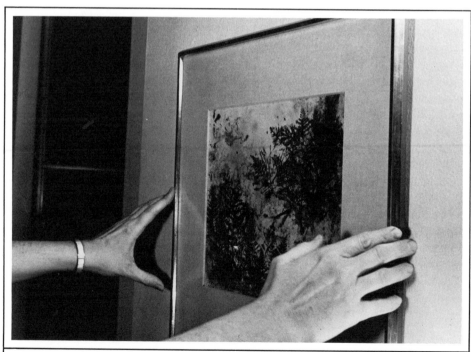

*Obsessive-compulsives are usually overly meticulous, the sort of people who cannot bear the sight of a lopsided picture or having anything in their physical environment even slightly out of place.*

population suffered from the disorder. In recent years mental-health experts have revised their thinking. The Epidemiologic Catchment Area Program estimated that 1.5% of adults in the United States suffer obsessive-compulsive disorder. More-over, studies by Judith Rapoport, M.D., at the National Insti-tute of Mental Health and others indicate that perhaps .3% of children and early adolescents are true obsessive-com-pulsives and that an even greater number show some symp-toms. Researchers now believe that around 2% of the population suffers from obsessive-compulsive behavior.

Rarely does a person suffer only a single obsession. Over time, an existing obsession may wane and be replaced by another. Most obsessions are simply absurd. But sometimes there is a grain of truth to them. Germs, indeed, do cause illnesses, and washing the hands and body can help prevent diseases. But even when an obsession has some truth to it, an obsessive-compulsive like Myra F. will carry it to a ridic-ulous extreme.

## *Characteristics of Obsession*

After reviewing three major studies of the symptoms found among people with obsessions, psychiatrists Donald W. Goodwin and Samuel B. Guze concluded in their book *Psychiatric Diagnosis* that the illness usually manifests itself in the form of one or more of these basic thought patterns:

•Obsessional ideas: Repeated, unwanted, and distressing thoughts that are obscene, blasphemous, or nonsensical in-terfere with the person's normal train of thinking.

•Obsessional images: Vivid and disturbing scenes of vio-lence, sex, or disgusting things (excrement, vomit, spilled blood) repeatedly come to mind.

•Obsessional convictions: These usually follow the illog-ical line of reasoning that a thought alone can have evil con-sequences. For example, a man might be obsessed with the idea that to think ill of his son will cause the child's death. Such thoughts may be both believed and disbelieved at the same time.

•Obsessional rumination: Obsessive-compulsives will sometimes engage in prolonged and inconclusive thinking about a topic that interferes with other thoughts. Often the obsessive thoughts focus on complex, unanswerable religious questions.

•Obsessional impulses: These involve fears of losing self-control. The afflicted person will harbor unwarranted concerns about becoming addicted to drugs or alcohol, inflicting self-injury, harming others — often a child or close relative — or doing some embarrassing act, such as screaming blasphemies or obscenities in church. There is no evidence, however, that obsessive-compulsive disorder makes a person more susceptible to violent or criminal behavior.

•Obsessional fears: These include distressing thoughts of illnesses, germs, dirt, personal injury, or performing bizarre acts.

•Obsessional rituals: These are obsessions in action. These acts, performed over and over again, are a visible manifestation of the obsessive thoughts occupying the mind. These rituals include such things as repeatedly counting the same objects — such as the number of pens on a desk; re-checking to see if something has been done — such as going back 10, 20, or 30 times to make sure the gas cooking stove has been turned off; and cleanliness rituals — compulsive showering, hand washing, and dusting.

Obsessive-compulsives are usually meticulous, indecisive, and ambivalent. They frequently will do something and then do it again and again, never quite satisfied it is right. They may count and recount the dollar bills in a cash drawer or arrange pens and pencils in a special order and then rearrange them in the same way. With such attention to detail, obsessive-compulsives generally do well in school — although some spend so much time on rituals that their studies suffer — and in jobs where precision and order are important. They tend, in fact, to be neatness freaks who always dress in proper attire and believe everything has its place and must be kept there. Yet many have a secret, segregated, and slovenly part of their lives, even if it is nothing more than a single drawer where clothes are tossed haphazardly. In addition, obsessive-compulsives are usually stubborn, a trait that can make them hard people to deal with and often difficult parents.

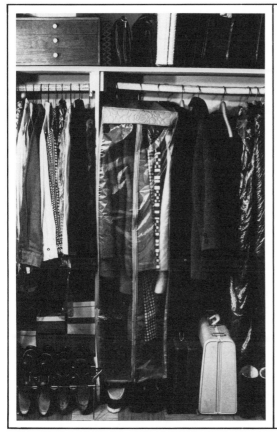

*A shipshape closet. Fanatical tidiness is the hallmark of the obsessive-compulsive's world. Needless to say, there is nothing wrong with being well organized, but an abnormal preoccupation with order can interfere with normal functioning.*

Many young children afflicted with obsessive-compulsive disorder consider the rituals that occupy so much of their lives as perfectly natural. However, older adolescents and adults realize that these rituals are not normal. Yet they continue to do them because it is the only way they can find relief from a deep sense of foreboding and apprehension. Some even harbor fears that some dreadful harm will befall them or someone they love if they do not perform the rituals.

Obsessive-compulsive behavior afflicts both sexes equally, although it appears to occur in males at an earlier average age, at least in children. The illness generally develops before age 25; fewer than 15% of cases occur after age 35. Rapoport has identified fully developed obsessive-compulsive symptoms in children as young as age six.

The disorder may strike suddenly, or it may come on gradually. The symptoms may be unremitting, or they may be episodic, going into partial or complete remission at times in a manner similar to primary depression. Even the most severe cases, however, tend to decrease gradually in intensity over many years.

The association of depression and obsessive-compulsive behavior has been recognized since at least 1896. Depressed people may suffer obsessions and compulsions. Obsessive-compulsives often develop mild, moderate, or even severe depression. The two disorders are so intertwined that it is difficult at times for psychiatrists to tell which disorder came first. Some experts have suggested that obsessive-compulsive disorder may be a variety of depression rather than a distinct illness in itself. The issue still remains open. In her studies Rapoport found that obsessive-compulsive children do not show the classic symptoms of depression.

The 19th-century German neurologist Karl Westphal coined the term "obsessional neurosis" for the mental disturbance officially known today as obsessive-compulsive dis-

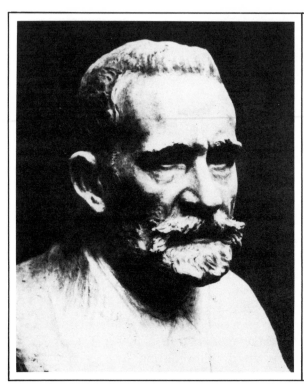

*Emile Kraepelin, the pioneering German psychologist. Both he and Freud used the term "obsessional neurosis" as a synonym for obsessive-compulsive behavior.*

order. Writers more than two centuries earlier had described the problem in considerable detail. Both Emil Kraepelin and Sigmund Freud used the term *obsessional neurosis* in their pioneering writings on psychiatric illnesses, and it remains a synonym today for obsessive-compulsive behavior. Freud described the ailment as follows: "The patient's mind is occupied with thoughts that do not really interest him, he feels impulses which seem alien to him, and he is impelled to perform actions which not only afford him no pleasure, but from which he is powerless to desist." Although Freud saw the illness as a purely psychological problem, as with a number of other mental illnesses, the question of whether obsessive-compulsive behavior results from nature, from nurture, or from an interaction of the two remains in dispute.

## What Causes Obsessive-Compulsive Behavior?

Freud envisioned the problem as related to deep-rooted conflicts and anxieties. The Freudian concept traces obsessive-compulsive problems back to the so-called anal phase of development, the time when a young child is being toilet trained. Until this time, the child has largely been allowed freedom. Now he is ordered by his parents to conform to unwanted rules. A battle of wills between parent and child ensues. Conflict develops as the child's attitude switches back and forth between compliance and stubborn resistance. It is well known that obsessive-compulsives can be as stubborn as the most hardheaded three year old.

Psychiatrists and psychologists who subscribe to learning theory see obsessional thinking as a conditioned or learned response to anxiety-provoking events. Compulsions develop when a person finds that the tension and fears associated with his obsessions lessen if he performs a certain act. This compulsion is reinforced each time the ritualistic act is performed and the tension diminishes.

Researchers have studied what factors within a family might cause or contribute to the development of the disorder. Studies suggest that the parents of obsessive-compulsives tend to be stubborn, unyielding, tightfisted with money, strong and strict in their religious beliefs, and demanding of their children. Many obsessive-compulsives remember being raised in homes with rigid rules and being told repeatedly

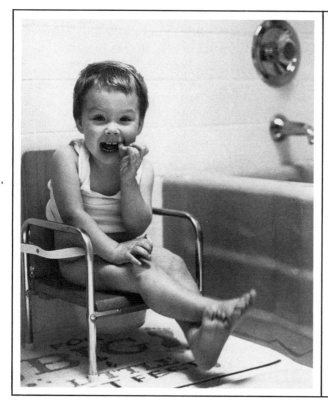

*Freudian theory holds that obsessive-compulsive disorders can be traced back to deep conflicts between parent and child during toilet training.*

what was good, what was bad, and how things in the world should be. Yet such characteristics are difficult to quantify with any precision. At this point, no one knows whether there is a pattern of parental behavior that plays some role in producing obsessive-compulsive disorder.

Partly because obsessive-compulsive behavior was considered rare for so long, researchers have not examined its possible genetic roots as closely as they have those of a number of other disorders. Evidence suggests that the illness runs in families. But does this mean that inherited genes play a role or that people develop the ailment because of their relationship with a parent who suffers from the disorder? Studies of twins show that if 1 identical twin has the disorder, 8 times out of 10 the other twin will be afflicted, as well. The problem is that all the twins in these studies were raised together rather than apart, and the findings again could be interpreted as resulting from either nature or nurture.

## Treating Obsessive-Compulsive Disorders

Reassurance is important in treating obsessive-compulsive behavior. People with the disorder need to be told it sometimes improves on its own and that it is highly unlikely that they will surrender to their impulses to cause harm or embarrass themselves. But obsessive-compulsives are notoriously resistant to psychotherapy, and talk alone rarely helps them. Indeed, the kind of insight therapies initiated by Sigmund Freud may even do more harm than good.

The most common treatment is exposure therapy. Similar to the technique (described in Chapter 4) used to treat some phobias, the patient is gradually exposed to the very thing he fears, under the careful guidance of a therapist. Someone terrified of germs might be asked to touch something soiled and eventually to make mud pies. Sometimes the patient is asked merely to imagine such a scene, but actually confronting the feared object appears to be more effective. During the exposure sessions, the therapist offers encouragement and reinforcement and may prevent the person from engaging in his ritual responses, such as hand washing. The patient may have as many as 30 such treatment sessions. This approach also requires a lot of work by patients on their own.

Physicians have tried treating obsessive-compulsives with a number of different drugs. With the exception of clomipramine, medications have not proved very helpful. Clomipramine is a tricyclic antidepressant sold widely in Europe and Canada, but used only experimentally in the United States at the time of this writing. Tests of the drug have found it is generally effective against obsessional thoughts. But study results are mixed on its effectiveness in reducing compulsive rituals. Moreover, there is some evidence that obsessive-compulsives who are not depressed may do equally well or better with exposure therapy.

Obsessive-compulsive behavior is a difficult disorder to treat. Even when therapy is successful, patients are not always pleased. Some find they do not know what to do with all the time they used to spend on their rituals. One research team testing clomipramine reported, "A few of our patients have indeed stopped taking the drug, stating that they actually preferred their rituals to an attempt to cope with the demands of an ordinary existence."

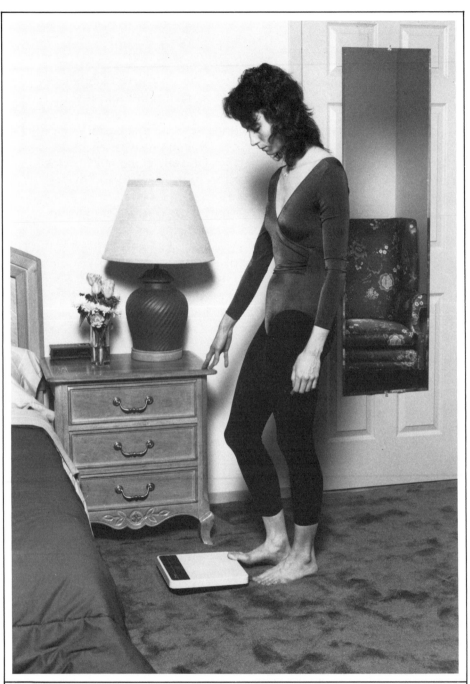

*Anorexia nervosa is a form of self-starvation motivated by an obsession with body image. Anorexics diet relentlessly but remain convinced that they are too heavy even when they have reached the point of emaciation.*

# CHAPTER 6

# ANOREXIA NERVOSA
# AND BULIMIA

Susan W.'s mother was delighted when her 15-year-old daughter decided to lose some weight. Susan was not fat, but both agreed that it would help Susan's appearance if she slimmed her thighs and flattened her stomach. So Susan began. She memorized the calorie counts of all the foods she ate and stopped eating the most fattening. She began exercising vigorously each day. In 3 months, Susan had lost more than 20 pounds, but insisted she was still too fat. In spite of her mother's pleas, the girl kept losing weight until she had dropped to 80 pounds. Her face was gaunt and her cheeks sunken, her arms and legs were thin sticks, and only skin seemed to cover her ribs, hips, and shoulder bones. Yet the girl still complained that she was overweight.

Susan was suffering from anorexia nervosa, a puzzling mental disturbance in which victims can actually starve themselves to death in the belief that they are too fat. The pop singer Karen Carpenter, who in 1983 died of heart complications caused by anorexia, is probably this eating disorder's most famous casualty.

In recent years, anorexia nervosa and bulimia, another eating disorder, have increasingly captured the attention of physicians and the public. Both tend to afflict adolescent girls or young women. Both disorders can have extremely serious

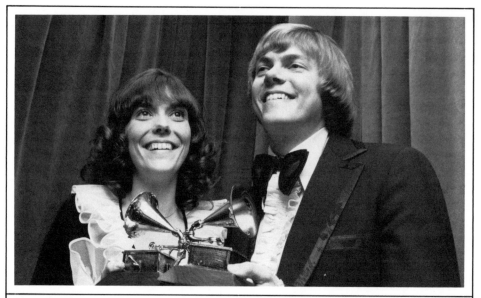

*The popular singing group The Carpenters display the Grammy award they won in 1972. Karen Carpenter was a victim of anorexia nervosa and died of heart failure—a complication of her illness—in 1983.*

physical consequences, including death. Both appear to be on the increase in the United States. Both are extraordinarily difficult to treat. The cause of each remains as baffling in the 20th century as when anorexia nervosa was first described nearly 500 years ago.

Anorexia nervosa is an intense fear of being fat that compels a person to diet relentlessly. Anorexics feel too fat even when emaciated. The word anorexia — which means loss of appetite — is misleading, because the anorexic's appetite does not disappear until late in the disease. The German word for the illness — *pubertaetsmagersucht*, "adolescent pursuit of thinness" — provides a more accurate description. The first medical description of anorexia nervosa was written by an Italian physician in 1500. In the centuries that followed, other doctors wrote from time to time of this odd and seemingly rare ailment.

Bulimia, which means "ox hunger," is an irresistible craving for food that leads to repeated episodes of binge eating — the ingestion of huge amounts of food within two hours or less. Bulimics do not stop gorging themselves until they suffer abdominal pain, fall asleep, or are interrupted by someone or something, such as a telephone call. Binge eating may be followed by self-induced vomiting to get rid of the excessive calories, and bulimics often fast between periods of binging. They are very much aware that their eating habits are abnormal, and they worry — even to the point of becoming depressed—about their uncontrolled consumption.

Until 1980, bulimia was regarded as a form of anorexia nervosa. Today the two conditions are classified as distinct disorders. A person may suffer one or the other, or both. Perhaps as many as half of all anorexics also go through bulimic binges during their illness.

### How Widespread Are Anorexia and Bulimia?

Little is known about just how common either eating disorder is. Precise incidence figures do not exist, and available estimates vary considerably. There is, however, wide agreement that anorexia nervosa and bulimia primarily affect white fe-

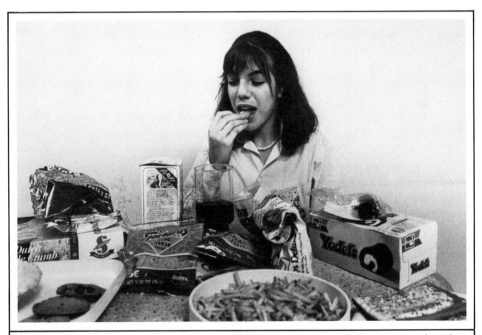

*Bulimia is an eating disorder characterized by a debilitating cycle of uncontrollable binge eating and purging.*

males. Indeed, girls and young women probably make up 90–95% of all anorexics. It is also widely believed that cases of bulimia and anorexia have increased dramatically since the late 1960s.

According to psychiatrists Donald W. Goodwin and Samuel B. Guze, data from community psychiatric centers in Scotland, England, and the United States suggest an annual incidence of one case of anorexia nervosa per 100,000 population. This would mean about 2,400 new cases in the United States each year. The Epidemiologic Catchment Area Program estimated that 1 in 1,000 Americans suffers anorexia sometime during their life. Other studies suggest .4% of teenage girls experience some degree of anorexia nervosa.

Even less is known about the incidence of bulimia. A survey by Harvard University psychiatrists suggests that between 2.2 and 7.6 million have or have had the disorder. A 1981 study at a New York college found that 13% of all students and 19% of female students were bulimic. A survey of more than 1,700 California high school sophomores by Stanford University researchers concluded in 1986 that up to 13% of teenagers suffer some degree of bulimia.

As mentioned earlier, anorexia nervosa almost always begins during the teen years, although the illness has struck as early as age 11 and as late as the fifties. As it did with Susan W., the disorder usually begins with concern about a mild weight problem. This legitimate concern then somehow turns into an intense fear of becoming fat and a distorted mental image of one's own body. Anorexia nervosa may exist as a single episode of progressive, debilitating weight loss extending for months or years. Or it may come and go — a bout of extreme dieting followed by a remission to normal or nearly normal eating, followed again by excessive food restrictions.

## Self-starvation

Anorexics often subsist on 600 calories a day. Those who binge and purge may consume 5,000 calories or more at a sitting but then vomit all but about 800 calories. Anorexics over 18, by medical definition, have lost 25% of their original body weight. Under 18, the diagnosis is applied if the excessive dieters are 25% below their projected weight on

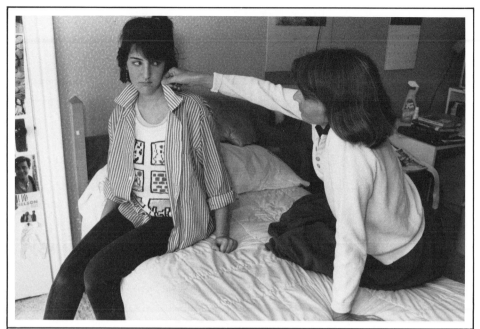

*A moody adolescent and her mother. Anorexia almost always strikes during the teenage years. It often begins with a concern about a mild weight problem that somehow turns into an intense fear of becoming fat.*

growth charts. The refusal to eat adequately can lead to malnutrition so severe that patients must be hospitalized to save their lives.

Although fear of their own body weight and a preoccupation with dieting dominate the thinking and conversations of anorexics, they rarely acknowledge that anything is amiss. Indeed, anorexics tend to be very chipper people — alert, cheerful, energetic, even hyperactive at times. Often they engage in strenuous exercise programs, an effective and socially acceptable way to keep very thin. But as the illness progresses, the typical anorexic increasingly isolates herself (Because the overwhelming majority of anorexics are women, the feminine pronoun will be used when referring to an anorexic) from family and friends.

The prolonged starvation associated with severe anorexia nervosa causes the breakdown of muscle throughout the body, including the heart. This causes the disorder's most tragic consequence — death. Follow-up studies of anorexics whose self-starvation required hospitalization have found that 10–21% of them died prematurely — that is, younger than would be expected. Starvation can damage heart muscle to the point of cardiac failure, or it may upset the body's important mineral balance and lead to abnormal heartbeats. Either can cause sudden death. Other common complications include amenorrhea — abnormal absence of menstruation — depression, and anxiety.

## The Binge-and-Purge Syndrome

Less is known about bulimia than anorexia nervosa. But severe bulimia is a potentially life-threatening condition. The mind's eye of the bulimic also distorts her body image. Most believe they are overweight, but this distorted self-portrait is not as severe as the anorexic's. Bulimics are usually of normal or near normal weight, although some may be 10–15% above or below their ideal. They do go through

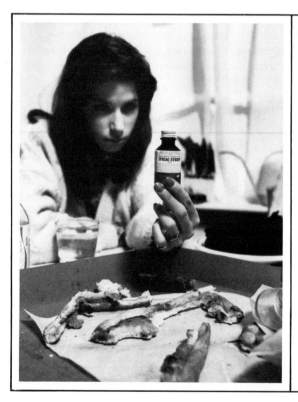

A bulimic prepares to swallow ipecac—a drug that induces vomiting.

frequent weight fluctuations of 10 pounds or more brought on by their habit of alternating food binges with fasts.

A bulimic may average anywhere from a food binge a week to more than 40. During these binges, they consume thousands of calories in an hour or two — as many as 55,000 in one documented instance. They often favor sweet, fattening foods that can be eaten quickly. Consider this "meal" consumed by a young woman in a single sitting: four tuna-fish sandwiches, three oranges, a quart of ice cream, and a chocolate cake, all washed down with a quart of diet soda.

After such gorgings, bulimics typically find themselves beset by guilt and depression. Many try to purge their bodies of the calories and fluids they have consumed with laxatives, diuretics ("water pills"), and enemas. A finger or some foreign object, such as a toothbrush, may be forced down the throat to induce vomiting. A few patients are known to have forced themselves to vomit 40 times in a day. There is considerable variation among bulimics, but typically, they gorge and purge a few times a day for several days. Then they stop for a time — often fasting during this period — before going back to binge eating.

Bulimics also face the danger of sudden death. The binge-purge pattern can damage almost any of the body's organs, including the heart and kidney. Vomiting can deplete the body of vital potassium — sometimes to the extent that the heart can no longer keep pumping. Abuse of the drug ipecac to induce vomiting may cause fatal heart-muscle damage or abnormal heartbeats. In a few rare cases, bulimics have engorged so much food that their stomachs have ruptured. Among the other complications of bulimia are inflamed lungs resulting from food particles being inhaled while vomiting, tooth damage and decay caused by stomach acids, and painful swelling of the salivary glands. Depression and anxiety are common among bulimics, and many have suicidal thoughts. But it remains unclear how many of these people attempt to take their own lives or how many succeed.

## What Causes Severe Eating Disorders?

Researchers in recent years have hotly pursued the cause or causes of anorexia nervosa and bulimia. But as yet no solid agreement has emerged about the disorder's origins. In the

Freudian tradition, one theory holds that anorexia nervosa represents a rejection of adult sexuality. But a more popular belief is that family dynamics — the interactions between the parents and the child from birth — play an important role in the onset of eating disorders. Food is, after all, a major factor in the parent-child relationship almost from the instant of birth. Somehow, one theory goes, the parent-child interaction produced inner conflicts that the child seeks to solve through manipulation of food.

The family situation has been more extensively analyzed in anorexia nervosa than in bulimia. Several studies have suggested that the parents of anorexics are controlling, demanding, overprotective, rigid, have problems resolving family conflicts, and are strongly attached to their children. A University of Wisconsin study reported that anorexic and bulimic young women viewed their parents as more blaming, rejecting, and neglectful of them than did women who did not suffer eating disorders. Many anorexics contend they have spent their lives trying unsuccessfully to live up to their parents' expectations. But no matter how much they accomplish, they are always made to feel they are second-best when compared to others.

Some authorities on eating disorders have suggested that the anorexic feels that she has been dominated and controlled by her parents as far back as she can remember. The child accepts this. To compensate, however, she eventually takes control of her eating habits, coming to dominate her food intake as thoroughly as her parents dominated her.

Such ideas remain theories, and they are not without their detractors, who claim that although the personality traits attributed to the parents of anorexics are common to many humans, anorexia is uncommon. In addition, researchers at the Johns Hopkins University School of Medicine have failed to find any signs of disturbed family relationships in fully 20% of their anorexic patients. So clearly there is more to the disorder than family interactions.

Whether eating disorders run in families or have a genetic component to them is unknown. Physical differences have been noted between those with eating disorders and those free of them. Studies have indicated that the hypothalamus, a major source of brain hormones, is impaired in anorexics. Some male anorexics appear to have low levels of

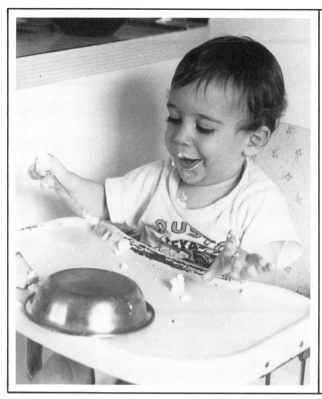

Some researchers maintain that severe eating disorders have their origins in early childhood, when mealtime becomes a battleground between parent and child.

the sex hormone testosterone. Whether these and other observed differences play a role in causing the disorder or are results of it remains unclear.

## Can These Disorders Be Treated?

At this time, there is no general agreement about how best to treat anorexia nervosa and bulimia. The two are difficult and frustrating for anyone involved in the process, whether parent or health professional. Success takes years, and far too often great effort ends only in failure. Getting patients to cooperate is a major problem in treating the two disorders, particularly anorexia nervosa. Anorexics often refuse to take drugs for fear that the medication will cause them to gain weight. Physicians and families have known for years that nothing they can do will force an anorexic to gain weight if she does not want to.

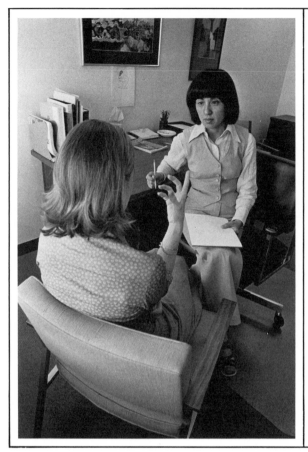

A therapist confers with her patient. Although there is no guaranteed cure for severe eating disorders, a number of new treatment approaches have begun to show promise.

As previously mentioned, severely malnourished anorexics require hospitalization to counteract their starvation. Sometimes this means feeding, even force-feeding the patient through a tube. Bulimics whose illness is not combined with anorexia usually do not need to be hospitalized.

However, treating the medical problems does nothing to correct the anorexic's psychological illness. Psychotherapy remains the main treatment for both anorexia and bulimia. Working one on one with a therapist or in a group with other patients can build feelings of competence and self-worth that will change the patient's distorted body image and obsession with dieting. Family therapy may alter relationships that contribute to the eating disorders. Behavioral therapy is often used. Anorexics may be rewarded with special privileges as they gain weight. One approach commonly used with bulimics is the "planned binge," during which the patient is asked to gorge herself as the therapist or a family member watches. This method can be quite effective, for many bulimics cannot consume gross amounts of food in public.

Drugs have not produced the same dramatic benefits in these two disorders as they have in many other mental disturbances. However, some bulimics treated with antidepressant drugs have shown sustained improvement. Some evidence suggests that the medications suppress the urge to binge even in bulimics who are not depressed. Antidepressant medications have proved less useful in treating anorexia nervosa, although some improvement has been reported in some cases. Efforts to treat anorexics with drugs that affect the hypothalamus have yielded inconclusive results. A few years ago, a Stanford University research team concluded that no treatment in the last 50 years has made a significant difference in the natural course of anorexia nervosa.

About half of all hospitalized anorexics suffer at least one relapse after their release. Studies indicate that only 35–50% of those hospitalized are eating normally 5 years later. Among bulimics, 50–60% are no longer bingers a year after treatment ends. Among both anorexics and bulimics, the shorter the duration of their illness before treatment, the better their chances are for a full recovery.

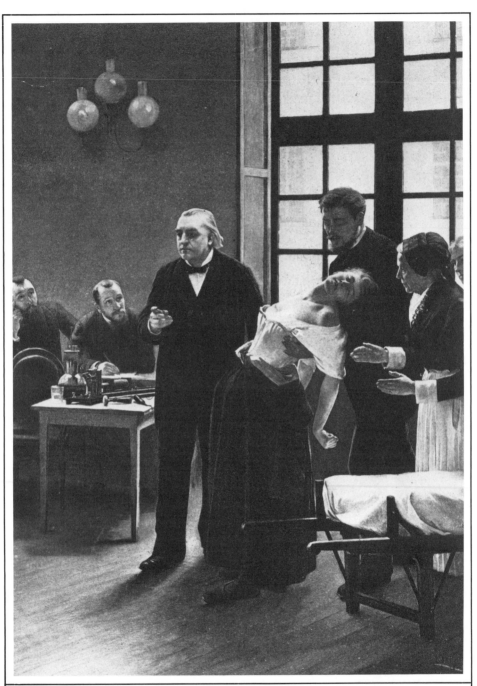

Jean M. Charcot, the great 19th-century French neurologist, lectures on a patient's condition. Charcot devoted the last years of his career to controversial studies of hysteria and hypnotism.

# CHAPTER 7

# HYSTERIA

**F**ew psychiatric conditions are as confounding to physicians as hysteria. It is a difficult disorder to recognize readily and a harder one still to treat successfully. Yet for these very reasons, and for its historical importance to modern psychiatry, hysteria remains a fascinating mental disturbance.

Hysteria — also known as somatization disorder and Briquet's syndrome — nearly always occurs in females. It is a pattern of behavior that centers around numerous physical complaints that are made often and are usually described in very dramatic terms. Yet despite their pain — and hysterics do suffer — there seems to be no organic basis for their symptoms. Hysterics go to doctors often, consume many different drugs in large quantities over the years, and have high hospitalization and surgery rates.

Their greatly varied symptoms, their obvious discomfort, and their habit of jumping from one doctor to another explain why hysteria can go undetected for many years. Although the disorder generally begins in the teenage years and rarely starts after the first two decades of life, hysterics typically are in their thirties before their problem is recognized. It is the multiple symptoms with no detectable cause that finally identify the hysteric, but usually not until she has been hospitalized and operated on a number of times.

Hysterics see themselves as sickly people. They believe that they have been ill a good part of their lives. By medical definition, a hysteric suffers from as many as 37 specific symptoms. Women must have described at least 14 of the symp-

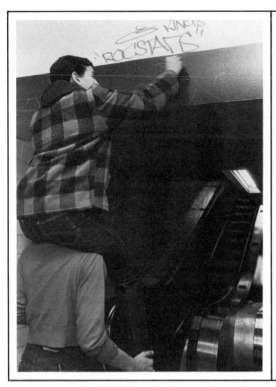

*A young man defaces a high-school building with graffiti. Interesting parallels have been drawn between hysteria, a condition that primarily afflicts females, and sociopathy, primarily a male disorder. A person with either disorder frequently has a history of delinquency or antisocial behavior going back to childhood and adolescence.*

toms over several years — and men at least 12 — before they are diagnosed with the disorder. Pain of one sort or another — in the back, chest, joints, fingers, toes, abdomen, genital area, and during urination — is a prominent complaint. So are shortness of breath, heart palpitations, dizziness, nausea, vomiting spells (other than during pregnancy), gas bloating, diarrhea, and problems in their sex life, including indifference, lack of pleasure, and pain during intercourse.

## Conversion Symptoms

The most dramatic symptoms seen in hysterics are called conversion symptoms, a group of unexplained problems that suggest serious neurological diseases. Unexplained simply means that no physical cause for them can be found. These symptoms include blindness, blurred vision, deafness, paralysis, muscle weakness, convulsions, amnesia, voice loss, fainting, and difficulty walking and urinating. Conversion symptoms are not unique to hysteria. Indeed, they occur independently of it, and they are found in some patients suffering from any of the psychiatric illnesses.

Nevertheless, conversion symptoms are considered classic to hysteria. They are dramatic and frightening, but usually easy to distinguish from a genuine organic ailment. In hysterical blindness, for example, the person reacts normally to light and will avoid a clear threat — a fist thrust quickly at her face. In hysterical paralysis, the person's reflexes remain normal. Such people are not faking their illness. They are, in fact, blind or paralyzed. However, the cause is psychological, not neurological. Thus their bodies retain functions that their minds will not allow them to use.

Everyone experiences many of the symptoms associated with hysteria during their lifetime. But when a doctor takes a medical history, there is a difference between how normal people and hysterics respond. Hysterics will frequently list all the symptoms they have ever experienced. People who are not hysterics stick to the specific symptoms that brought them to the doctor. They do not bother describing a dizzy spell or racing heart from years before. The physician whose patient reveals a great number of symptoms from a wide range of body systems — often in a colorful and dramatic way — is likely to be talking with a hysteric.

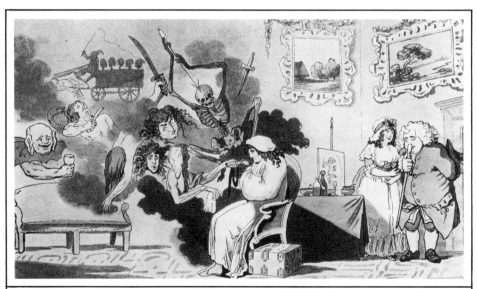

The Hypochondriac, *an 18th-century engraving. Hysterics are plagued by maladies for which no physical cause can be found.*

Hysterics are usually highly emotional and sentimental people, and their lives tend to be chaotic. They frequently marry men who are totally unsuited to them. And when the marriage ends in divorce, they plunge into matrimony again with an equally unsuitable male.

Hysteria is not a frequent mental disturbance, but just how common it is remains unsettled. The Epidemiologic Catchment Area Program estimated that .1% of American adults suffer hysteria at any one time. Other studies have suggested that perhaps as many as 1% of adult American women are hysterics. Nonetheless, the term hysteric is too often applied indiscriminately and inaccurately, by laymen and physicians alike.

Hysteria was first recognized some 4,000 years ago, apparently in ancient Egypt. The name itself has been used since at least the 4th century B.C. It comes from the ancient Greek word for uterus and reflects the belief of the time that hysteria resulted from a womb having shifted from its proper position. In 1859 the French physician P. Briquet initiated the modern practice of diagnosing hysteria by a particular pattern of symptoms and signs.

Hysteria fascinated Sigmund Freud at the time he was formulating psychoanalysis. Several of his early patients suffered symptoms of the disorder, and they responded dramatically to Freud's talking cure. Much of his therapeutic technique evolved from this experience, and Freud expanded it to other psychiatric illnesses. In a sense, the master psychiatrist was fortunate that his first patients were hysterics, for other mental disorders — to one degree or another — proved less responsive to psychoanalysis.

No other psychiatric disturbance so neatly fits Freud's theory that repressing unconscious sexual impulses creates conflicts that manifest themselves in mental illnesses. Freudians view hysteria as a simulated illness that reflects the subconscious mind's attempt to work out unconscious conflicts. The illness provides the hysteric the secondary gain of sympathy and support from family and friends and allows her to shirk duties and responsibilities she finds distasteful. Conversion symptoms, according to Freudian theory, stem from the repression of some single, emotionally disturbing event — the first sight of the male penis is often cited as an example. The event is buried in the subconscious. But when the event recurs, the person responds by converting the emotional response into a physical symptom — blindness, deafness, paralysis. This blocks out the emotionally disturbing experience.

## Family and Gender

Hysteria does run in families. About one in five of the parents, siblings, and children of hysterics also suffers hysteria. It is unknown whether this family history means the disorder is inherited or whether hysterics raise their children to be hysterics. One study of adopted children found that those who had a biological parent who was a hysteric were far more likely to suffer hysteria than those who did not have a hysterical natural parent. This hints that inheritance plays a role in the disorder, but it is far from conclusive proof.

Researchers have noted some interesting similarities between hysteria — predominantly a disorder of females — and sociopathy, a pattern of repeated antisocial, delinquent, and criminal behavior primarily found in males. Sociopathy — often called antisocial personality — begins in childhood or early adolescence. Those with the disorder frequently get into trouble with the police and other authorities, to the detriment of their family and social relationships, schooling, job, and marriage.

Many women with hysteria have a history of delinquency or antisocial behavior as young girls and teens. Female criminals often appear to suffer a mixture of hysteria and sociopathy. Conversion symptoms — which may accompany any psychiatric illness — occur most often in two disorders: hysteria and sociopathy. In addition, the fathers, brothers, and sons of hysterics are more likely to be sociopathic than the close male relatives of people who are not hysterics. This evidence has led to the suggestion that perhaps hysteria and sociopathy share the same underlying cause — but for some unknown reason different disorders occur in the two sexes.

Treating a hysteric is, with rare exceptions, an exercise in frustration and futility. Physicians in ancient Egypt — following the belief that the symptoms of hysteria resulted from a wandering womb — sought to attract the uterus back to its proper place with sweet-smelling substances. Physicians today fare little better in curing hysterics than did their colleagues in the time of the pharaohs. Hysterics are notoriously

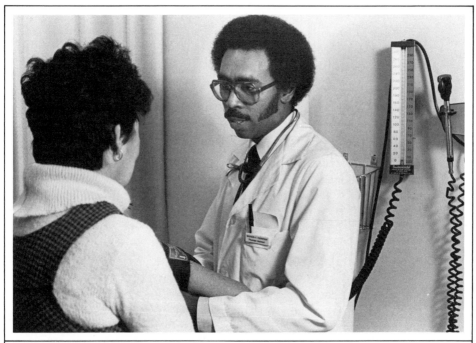

*A woman patient consults with her physician. Hysterics go to doctors often, consume many different drugs in large quantities over the years, and have high hospitalization and surgery rates.*

difficult to treat. They are manipulative and often play one therapist off against another, or they may provoke an argument between their therapist and their regular physician. Few hysterics willingly remain under a psychiatrist's care for long. As a result, dealing with these patients often falls to other physicians.

There are two advantages to diagnosing hysteria. First, the physician can be sure in at least 9 out of 10 cases that the symptoms will continue throughout life. Second, when the person does not fully fit the hysteria pattern, the physician can feel fairly confident that in most cases some physical ailment will eventually emerge to explain the symptoms. Either piece of information will help guide the doctor in dealing with the patient.

If the patient is a true hysteric, a major goal is to prevent the disorder's major complications. These include repeated surgical operations, getting hooked on prescription pain-killers and other drugs, marital problems and divorce, and suicide attempts. Hysterics are prone to attempt suicide, but only rarely do they actually kill themselves. Nonetheless, even a halfhearted suicide gesture can go awry and end in death. The key is to substitute psychological help and support — to the extent that the physician can — for medical treatment, which can do more harm than good. At the same time, the doctor must remain alert for signs of genuine physical illness. Hysterics do develop ulcers, heart disease, cancer, and all the other illnesses that afflict humans.

## Mass Hysteria

An intriguing and uncommon condition akin to the hysteria seen in individuals is mass hysteria. It is a dramatic event that never fails to attract wide attention when it strikes.

On the morning of May 21, 1979, 224 students at an elementary school in the Boston suburb of Norwood, Massachusetts, gathered for their final assembly of the year. Suddenly, a sixth-grade boy fainted. Within a short time one-third of the student body became ill. Doctors and ambulances rushed to the school. Thirty-four children were hospitalized with symptoms that included severe dizziness, weakness, hyperventilation (rapid, excessive breathing), headaches, nausea, and abdominal pain. Nearly 50 more were treated on the school grounds. Fortunately, none of the children suffered lasting ill effects.

Public-health investigators quickly began searching for contaminated food or water or for toxic chemicals that might have caused the sudden illnesses. They finally concluded that the children of Norwood had not been felled by some germ or poison but by a psychological epidemic—mass hysteria.

Mass hysteria involves a set of physical symptoms — the ones seen in the Norwood students — that affect a group of people, each of whom suffers at least one of the symptoms. The symptoms spread as if an epidemic were sweeping the group, and although they usually disappear quickly, relapses may occur. The symptoms suggest an unknown physical illness. In fact, the cause is psychological.

The disorder is uncommon — fewer than 50 episodes have been reported in English-language medical journals in this century — and puzzling. Like individual hysteria, mass hysteria primarily affects females. Sometimes the episodes are bizarre. In the 1970s, some women at a Malaysian computer-chip plant reported seeing demons when they looked through the microscopes they used in their work.

Because so few episodes of mass hysteria have been thoroughly studied, much remains unknown about the disorder. Over the past two decades, some progress has been made. Certainly fear and the power of suggestion play roles in the spread of the symptoms from one group member to others. Psychological stress — particularly a fear or feared loss — appears to be a key factor. At Norwood, for example, the school's well-liked principal was leaving; the sixth-grade class was graduating and leaving its old school for a new one; and the class had scheduled a trip, which for some members would be their first time away from home without their parents. Similarly, in 1973, 36 members of an Alabama high school band were hospitalized with dizziness, hyperventilation, headaches, or nausea. Heat may have been one factor, but another appears to be that the school was losing a game it expected to win easily.

Although stress appears important, not everyone has to be suffering the same stress. Many individuals may be experiencing many different forms of stress. When the right combination of events occurs, they react with the physical symptoms of mass hysteria. The first person to show signs of illness may not even feel stressed. Indeed, this person may be suffering from influenza or some other germ-caused disease. But his symptoms, in the right psychological setting, can trigger mass hysteria.

According to one theory, the stress must be high, and people must feel they are trapped in a situation they cannot escape. This would explain why so many mass-hysteria incidents in this century have occurred among schoolchildren and factory workers. Both must show up daily and spend time in a place where they may not want to be. Factory workers need their paychecks, and students are under pressure from their parents and society to attend school. One way to escape the stress of feeling trapped is to become ill.

This provides, in psychological terms, two "gains." First, the person escapes the stress, at least temporarily. Second, other people offer support. They tend the stricken individual; they provide encouragement; they give the person the sense of being loved by other humans. Some evidence suggests that a feeling of being isolated or ignored on the job or in school may help precipitate mass hysteria.

Psychologist Michael J. Colligan of the National Institute of Occupational Safety and Health found in testing people involved in mass hysteria episodes that those who became ill were more introverted and more depressed than those who did not. Moreover, they tend to be dependent, suggestible, and overly dramatic — behaviors typical of hysterics. Harvard psychiatrists Gary W. Small and Armand M. Nicholi, Jr., found a notable difference between those stricken Norwood students who required hospitalization and those who were treated at the school but not taken to the hospital. The hospitalized students had significantly higher rates of divorce and the death of a parent in their families. Such loss may make children more likely to be stressed by other losses, the two psychiatrists suggested. This may make them more vulnerable to mass hysteria.

No one knows if mass hysteria creates any long-term adverse effects. But at this time there is no evidence from short-term studies that such an experience causes lasting physical or psychological harm.

## Conclusion

The 20th century has witnessed revolutionary advances in the diagnosis and treatment of mental illnesses. Research into the workings of the brain has led to the development of psychiatric drugs that mitigate symptoms ranging from mild anxiety to severe disturbance. In assessing the progress science is making in this area, it is important to remember that only a few hundred years ago victims of mental illness were routinely subjected to lifelong confinement in dungeonlike facilities, sometimes were kept in chains, and frequently were the victims of superstition and persecution. To be sure, there is no magic cure in sight that would eliminate the waste and suffering wrought by diseases of the mind. Still, there is more movement in this direction now than in any previous era. This represents not only scientific progress but moral progress, as well.

# APPENDIX I

| Phobias | | | |
|---|---|---|---|
| **Name** | **Fear** | **Name** | **Fear** |
| acrophobia | high places | murophobia | mice |
| aerophobia | flying | mysophobia | dirt |
| ailurophobia | cats | nyctophobia | darkness |
| anthophobia | flowers and blossoms | ochlophobia | crowds |
| arachnophobia | spiders | ophidiophobia | snakes |
| belonophobia | needles | ornithophobia | birds |
| claustrophobia | small, enclosed spaces | phonophobia | telephones |
| cynophobia | dogs | porphyrophobia | purple |
| eremophobia | quiet, stillness | pyrophobia | fire |
| geniophobia | chins | rattusphobia | rats |
| gephyrophobia | bridges | siderodromophobia | railroads |
| graphobia | writing | spheksophobia | wasps |
| gynophobia | women | taphaphobia | being buried alive |
| herpetophobia | reptiles | thalassophobia | the sea |
| hypnophobia | sleep | trichophobia | hair |
| iophobia | rust | trypanophobia | drug injections |
| mikrophobia | germs | xenophobia | foreigners or strangers |

# APPENDIX II

## State Agencies
## for the Prevention and Treatment
## of Drug Abuse

**ALABAMA**
Department of Mental Health
Division of Mental Illness and
    Substance Abuse Community
    Programs
200 Interstate Park Drive
P.O. Box 3710
Montgomery, AL 36193
(205) 271-9253

**ALASKA**
Department of Health and Social
    Services
Office of Alcoholism and Drug
    Abuse
Pouch H-05-F
Juneau, AK 99811
(907) 586-6201

**ARIZONA**
Department of Health Services
Division of Behavioral Health
    Services
Bureau of Community Services
Alcohol Abuse and Alcoholism
    Section
2500 East Van Buren
Phoenix, AZ 85008
(602) 255-1238

Department of Health Services
Division of Behavioral Health
    Services
Bureau of Community Services
Drug Abuse Section
2500 East Van Buren
Phoenix, AZ 85008
(602) 255-1240

**ARKANSAS**
Department of Human Services
Office of Alcohol and Drug Abuse
    Prevention
1515 West 7th Avenue
Suite 310
Little Rock, AR 72202
(501) 371-2603

**CALIFORNIA**
Department of Alcohol and Drug
    Abuse
111 Capitol Mall
Sacramento, CA 95814
(916) 445-1940

**COLORADO**
Department of Health
Alcohol and Drug Abuse Division
4210 East 11th Avenue
Denver, CO 80220
(303) 320-6137

**CONNECTICUT**
Alcohol and Drug Abuse
    Commission
999 Asylum Avenue
3rd Floor
Hartford, CT 06105
(203) 566-4145

**DELAWARE**
Division of Mental Health
Bureau of Alcoholism and Drug
    Abuse
1901 North Dupont Highway
Newcastle, DE 19720
(302) 421-6101

**DISTRICT OF COLUMBIA**
Department of Human Services
Office of Health Planning and
  Development
601 Indiana Avenue, NW
Suite 500
Washington, D.C. 20004
(202) 724-5641

**FLORIDA**
Department of Health and
  Rehabilitative Services
Alcoholic Rehabilitation Program
1317 Winewood Boulevard
Room 187A
Tallahassee, FL 32301
(904) 488-0396

Department of Health and
  Rehabilitative Services
Drug Abuse Program
1317 Winewood Boulevard
Building 6, Room 155
Tallahassee, FL 32301
(904) 488-0900

**GEORGIA**
Department of Human Resources
Division of Mental Health and
  Mental Retardation
Alcohol and Drug Section
618 Ponce De Leon Avenue, NE
Atlanta, GA 30365-2101
(404) 894-4785

**HAWAII**
Department of Health
Mental Health Division
Alcohol and Drug Abuse Branch
1250 Punch Bowl Street
P.O. Box 3378
Honolulu, HI 96801
(808) 548-4280

**IDAHO**
Department of Health and Welfare
Bureau of Preventive Medicine
Substance Abuse Section
450 West State
Boise, ID 83720
(208) 334-4368

**ILLINOIS**
Department of Mental Health and
  Developmental Disabilities
Division of Alcoholism
160 North La Salle Street
Room 1500
Chicago, IL 60601
(312) 793-2907

Illinois Dangerous Drugs
  Commission
300 North State Street
Suite 1500
Chicago, IL 60610
(312) 822-9860

**INDIANA**
Department of Mental Health
Division of Addiction Services
429 North Pennsylvania Street
Indianapolis, IN 46204
(317) 232-7816

**IOWA**
Department of Substance Abuse
505 5th Avenue
Insurance Exchange Building
Suite 202
Des Moines, IA 50319
(515) 281-3641

**KANSAS**
Department of Social Rehabilitation
Alcohol and Drug Abuse Services
2700 West 6th Street
Biddle Building
Topeka, KS 66606
(913) 296-3925

**KENTUCKY**
Cabinet for Human Resources
Department of Health Services
Substance Abuse Branch
275 East Main Street
Frankfort, KY 40601
(502) 564-2880

**LOUISIANA**
Department of Health and Human
  Resources
Office of Mental Health and
  Substance Abuse
655 North 5th Street
P.O. Box 4049
Baton Rouge, LA 70821
(504) 342-2565

**MAINE**
Department of Human Services
Office of Alcoholism and Drug
  Abuse Prevention
Bureau of Rehabilitation
32 Winthrop Street
Augusta, ME 04330
(207) 289-2781

**MARYLAND**
Alcoholism Control Administration
201 West Preston Street
Fourth Floor
Baltimore, MD 21201
(301) 383-2977

State Health Department
Drug Abuse Administration
201 West Preston Street
Baltimore, MD 21201
(301) 383-3312

**MASSACHUSETTS**
Department of Public Health
Division of Alcoholism
755 Boylston Street
Sixth Floor
Boston, MA 02116
(617) 727-1960

Department of Public Health
Division of Drug Rehabilitation
600 Washington Street
Boston, MA 02114
(617) 727-8617

**MICHIGAN**
Department of Public Health
Office of Substance Abuse Services
3500 North Logan Street
P.O. Box 30035
Lansing, MI 48909
(517) 373-8603

**MINNESOTA**
Department of Public Welfare
Chemical Dependency Program
  Division
Centennial Building
658 Cedar Street
4th Floor
Saint Paul, MN 55155
(612) 296-4614

**MISSISSIPPI**
Department of Mental Health
Division of Alcohol and Drug Abuse
1102 Robert E. Lee Building
Jackson, MS 39201
(601) 359-1297

**MISSOURI**
Department of Mental Health
Division of Alcoholism and Drug
  Abuse
2002 Missouri Boulevard
P.O. Box 687
Jefferson City, MO 65102
(314) 751-4942

**MONTANA**
Department of Institutions
Alcohol and Drug Abuse Division
1539 11th Avenue
Helena, MT 59620
(406) 449-2827

**NEBRASKA**
Department of Public Institutions
Division of Alcoholism and Drug
Abuse
801 West Van Dorn Street
P.O. Box 94728
Lincoln, NB 68509
(402) 471-2851, Ext. 415

**NEVADA**
Department of Human Resources
Bureau of Alcohol and Drug Abuse
505 East King Street
Carson City, NV 89710
(702) 885-4790

**NEW HAMPSHIRE**
Department of Health and Welfare
Office of Alcohol and Drug Abuse
   Prevention
Hazen Drive
Health and Welfare Building
Concord, NH 03301
(603) 271-4627

**NEW JERSEY**
Department of Health
Division of Alcoholism
129 East Hanover Street CN 362
Trenton, NJ 08625
(609) 292-8949

Department of Health
Division of Narcotic and Drug
   Abuse Control
129 East Hanover Street CN 362
Trenton, NJ 08625
(609) 292-8949

**NEW MEXICO**
Health and Environment Department
Behavioral Services Division
Substance Abuse Bureau
725 Saint Michaels Drive
P.O. Box 968
Santa Fe, NM 87503
(505) 984-0020, Ext. 304

**NEW YORK**
Division of Alcoholism and Alcohol
   Abuse
194 Washington Avenue
Albany, NY 12210
(518) 474-5417

Division of Substance Abuse
   Services
Executive Park South
Box 8200
Albany, NY 12203
(518) 457-7629

**NORTH CAROLINA**
Department of Human Resources
Division of Mental Health, Mental
   Retardation and Substance Abuse
   Services
Alcohol and Drug Abuse Services
325 North Salisbury Street
Albemarle Building
Raleigh, NC 27611
(919) 733-4670

**NORTH DAKOTA**
Department of Human Services
Division of Alcoholism and Drug
   Abuse
State Capitol Building
Bismarck, ND 58505
(701) 224-2767

**OHIO**
Department of Health
Division of Alcoholism
246 North High Street
P.O. Box 118
Columbus, OH 43216
(614) 466-3543

Department of Mental Health
Bureau of Drug Abuse
65 South Front Street
Columbus, OH 43215
(614) 466-9023

**OKLAHOMA**
Department of Mental Health
Alcohol and Drug Programs
4545 North Lincoln Boulevard
Suite 100 East Terrace
P.O. Box 53277
Oklahoma City, OK 73152
(405) 521-0044

**OREGON**
Department of Human Resources
Mental Health Division
Office of Programs for Alcohol and
    Drug Problems
2575 Bittern Street, NE
Salem, OR 97310
(503) 378-2163

**PENNSYLVANIA**
Department of Health
Office of Drug and Alcohol
    Programs
Commonwealth and Forster Avenues
Health and Welfare Building
P.O. Box 90
Harrisburg, PA 17108
(717) 787-9857

**RHODE ISLAND**
Department of Mental Health,
    Mental Retardation and Hospitals
Division of Substance Abuse
Substance Abuse Administration
    Building
Cranston, RI 02920
(401) 464-2091

**SOUTH CAROLINA**
Commission on Alcohol and Drug
    Abuse
3700 Forest Drive
Columbia, SC 29204
(803) 758-2521

**SOUTH DAKOTA**
Department of Health
Division of Alcohol and Drug Abuse
523 East Capitol, Joe Foss Building
Pierre, SD 57501
(605) 773-4806

**TENNESSEE**
Department of Mental Health and
    Mental Retardation
Alcohol and Drug Abuse Services
505 Deaderick Street
James K. Polk Building,
    Fourth Floor
Nashville, TN 37219
(615) 741-1921

**TEXAS**
Commission on Alcoholism
809 Sam Houston State Office
    Building
Austin, TX 78701
(512) 475-2577
Department of Community Affairs
Drug Abuse Prevention Division
2015 South Interstate Highway 35
P.O. Box 13166
Austin, TX 78711
(512) 443-4100

**UTAH**
Department of Social Services
Division of Alcoholism and Drugs
150 West North Temple
Suite 350
P.O. Box 2500
Salt Lake City, UT 84110
(801) 533-6532

**VERMONT**
Agency of Human Services
Department of Social and
    Rehabilitation Services
Alcohol and Drug Abuse Division
103 South Main Street
Waterbury, VT 05676
(802) 241-2170

**VIRGINIA**
Department of Mental Health and
   Mental Retardation
Division of Substance Abuse
109 Governor Street
P.O. Box 1797
Richmond, VA 23214
(804) 786-5313

**WASHINGTON**
Department of Social and Health
   Service
Bureau of Alcohol and Substance
   Abuse
Office Building—44 W
Olympia, WA 98504
(206) 753-5866

**WEST VIRGINIA**
Department of Health
Office of Behavioral Health Services
Division on Alcoholism and Drug
   Abuse
1800 Washington Street East
Building 3 Room 451
Charleston, WV 25305
(304) 348-2276

**WISCONSIN**
Department of Health and Social
   Services
Division of Community Services
Bureau of Community Programs
Alcohol and Other Drug Abuse
   Program Office
1 West Wilson Street
P.O. Box 7851
Madison, WI 53707
(608) 266-2717

**WYOMING**
Alcohol and Drug Abuse Programs
Hathaway Building
Cheyenne, WY 82002
(307) 777-7115, Ext. 7118

**GUAM**
Mental Health & Substance Abuse
   Agency
P.O. Box 20999
Guam 96921

**PUERTO RICO**
Department of Addiction Control
   Services
Alcohol Abuse Programs
P.O. Box B-Y Rio Piedras Station
Rio Piedras, PR 00928
(809) 763-5014

Department of Addiction Control
   Services
Drug Abuse Programs
P.O. Box B-Y Rio Piedras Station
Rio Piedras, PR 00928
(809) 764-8140

**VIRGIN ISLANDS**
Division of Mental Health,
   Alcoholism & Drug Dependency
   Services
P.O. Box 7329
Saint Thomas, Virgin Islands 00801
(809) 774-7265

**AMERICAN SAMOA**
LBJ Tropical Medical Center
Department of Mental Health Clinic
Pago Pago, American Samoa 96799

**TRUST TERRITORIES**
Director of Health Services
Office of the High Commissioner
Saipan, Trust Territories 96950

# Further Reading

Goodwin, Donald W., M.D. *Phobia: The Facts*. New York: Oxford University Press, 1983.

Goodwin, Donald W., M.D., and Samuel B. Guze, M.D. *Psychiatric Diagnosis*. New York: Oxford University Press, 1984.

Harris, Robert T., M.D. "The Perils of Gorging and Purging." *Acute Care Medicine*, April 1984, 15–17.

Herbert, Wray. "An Epidemic in the Works (Mass Hysteria)." *Science News*. 122 (September 18, 1982): 188–190.

Miller, Milton H., M.D. *If the Patient Is You (Or Someone You Love)*. New York: Scribners, 1977.

Sheehan, David V., M.D. *The Anxiety Disease*. New York: Scribners, 1983.

Snyder, Solomon H., M.D. *The Troubled Mind: A Guide to Release from Distress*. New York: McGraw-Hill, 1976.

Torrey, E. Fuller, M.D. *Surviving Schizophrenia*. New York: Harper & Row, 1983.

Travis, Carol. "Coping with Anxiety." *Science Digest*, February 1986, 46–50, 80–81.

Trubo, Richard. "Eating Disorders." *Medical World News*, July 9, 1984, 38–52.

Tsuang, Ming T. *Schizophrenia: The Facts*. New York: Oxford University Press, 1982.

Waldrop, M. Mitchell. "Youth Suicide: New Research Focuses on a Growing Social Problem." *Science*. 233 (August 22, 1986): 839–841.

Winokur, George, M.D. *Depression: The Facts*. New York: Oxford University Press, 1981.

Young, Patrick. "Americans Face Age of Anxiety." *Staten Island [NY] Advance*. January 24, 1987.

———. "Don't Panic! Doctors Offer Solutions for the No. 1 Problem." *The Mobile [AL] Press*. September 30, 1986.

———. "Scientists Seek Suicide Cure." *Saginaw [MI] News*. April 27, 1986.

# Glossary

**addiction** a condition caused by repeated drug use, characterized by a compulsive urge to continue using the drug, a tendency to increase the dosage, and physiological and/or psychological dependence

**affective illness** any of the disorders involving mood distortions, such as depression and manic-depressive illness

**agoraphobia** a phobic disorder in which a person avoids being alone or in public places for fear escape would be difficult in case of a sudden, incapacitating panic attack

**anorexia nervosa** an eating disorder found primarily in young females involving a distorted body image leading to relentless, sometimes fatal dieting

**antipsychotic** a class of drugs used to treat schizophrenia

**anxiety** a state of distress and uneasiness

**bipolar depression** a mental disorder in which people experience mood swings from highs to lows or suffer mania (highs) only

**bulimia** a condition characterized by eating enormous quantities, often followed by self-induced vomiting to purge the body

**catatonic schizophrenia** a category of schizophrenia characterized by abnormal body behaviors that range from almost complete immobility to frenzied motion

**chromosome** threadlike structures in each cell that contain the genes determining an organism's inherited traits

**compulsion** a repetitive act carried out as the result of an obsession

**concordance** the existence of one or more genetic traits in both members of a pair of twins

**conversion symptoms** dramatic symptoms such as blindness, deafness, paralysis, convulsions, and amnesia that suggest serious neurological disease, but for which no physical cause can be found

**delusions** false beliefs that are contrary to logic and reason

**depression** the most common of the serious mental illnesses, characterized by low moods extending over months, often with a sense of worthlessness and hopelessness

**dopamine** a neurotransmitter in the brain involved in emotional regulation and the control of body movement

**dysthymia** an affective illness in which symptoms of depression are present but with less severity

**electroconvulsive therapy** treatment, primarily for depression, involving brief pulses of electricity passed through the brain

**endogenous depression** "inner" depression that appears to rise from within and may occur without any stressful event

**exogenous depression** "outer" depression that appears triggered specifically by a stressful event

**exposure therapies** techniques in which phobics are exposed to the things they fear either gradually or with full intensity, so as to eliminate the fear

**generalized anxiety disorder** persistent severe anxiety that lasts at least one month

**hallucination** a sensory impression that has no basis in reality

**hebephrenic schizophrenia** a category of schizophrenia, characterized by pathetic attempts at comical behavior

**hysteria** a mental disorder in which patients report many medical symptoms for which no physical cause can be found

**lithium** a drug used to treat manic-depressive illness

**mania** a mood disorder characterized by euphoria, hyperactivity, intense excitement, and a surge of disjointed ideas

**manic-depressive illness** a mental disturbance in which a person's moods alternate between very high (mania) and very low (depression)

**mass hysteria** a set of symptoms — physical in nature but psychological in cause — that affect a number of people gathered together

**monoamine oxidase inhibitors** a group of drugs used to treat depression

**neurotransmitters** chemicals that help transmit signals from one nerve cell to another

**obsessive-compulsive disorder** a condition characterized by chronic obsessions that cause great mental distress and interfere with daily life; also, obsessional neurosis

**panic attack** a sudden sense of foreboding or terror accompanied by intense physical symptoms such as rapid breathing and heart rate, blurred vision, chest pains, and dizziness

**panic disorder** a chronic mental illness characterized by recurrent panic attacks

**paranoid schizophrenia** a category of schizophrenia, characterized by anxiety, anger, violent behavior, and delusions of persecution or grandeur

**phobia** an excessive, recurrent, and irrational fear that compels avoidance of a specific object, activity, or situation

**physical dependence** an adaption of the body to the presence of a drug such that its absence produces withdrawal symptoms

**primary depression** depression that occurs in someone who has never suffered another form of mental illness

**psychoanalysis** a method of treating mental disorders through the detection and analysis of usually subconscious feelings or conflicts

**psychological dependence** a condition in which the user craves a drug to maintain a sense of well-being and feels discomfort when deprived of it

**psychotherapy** "talking treatments"; a general term for a number of approaches that use mental rather than physical techniques to treat mental and emotional illnesses

**schizoaffective** a mental illness with the features of both schizophrenia and depression

**schizophrenia** a mental disorder in which a person loses touch with reality; characterized by a profound emotional withdrawal and bizarre behavior; often includes delusions and hallucinations

**schizophreniform** a schizoaffective illness with symptoms lasting more than a week, but less than six months

**secondary depression** depression that follows another mental illness

**social phobia** a persistent, irrational fear that compels a person to avoid an activity in public, such as speaking or eating

**sociopathy** antisocial personality; a mental disorder seen primarily in males that is characterized by repeated antisocial, delinquent, and criminal behavior

**tolerance** a decrease in susceptibility to the effects of a drug due to its continued administration, resulting in the user's need to increase the drug dosage in order to achieve the effects experienced previously

**tricyclic antidepressants** the most commonly prescribed group of drugs for depression

**unipolar depression** a mental disorder in which only low moods are experienced

**withdrawal** the physiological and psychological effects of the discontinued use of a drug

## PICTURE CREDITS

# Index

**Patrick Young** is a science and medical correspondent for the Newhouse News Service in Washington, D.C., and has explored the world and work of scientists and physicians for nearly two decades. In 1979, he served on the senior staff of the presidential commission that investigated the nuclear power plant accident at Three Mile Island. He is the author of *Drugs & Pregnancy* in Series 2 of the Encyclopedia of Psychoactive Drugs, published by Chelsea House. He has won over a dozen other national awards for his articles on medicine, the physical sciences, and space.

**Solomon H. Snyder,** M.D., is Distinguished Service Professor of Neuroscience, Pharmacology and Psychiatry at The Johns Hopkins University School of Medicine. He has served as president of the Society for Neuroscience and in 1978 received the Albert Lasker Award in Medical Research. He has authored *Uses of Marijuana, Madness and the Brain, The Troubled Mind, Biological Aspects of Mental Disorder,* and edited *Perspective in Neuropharmacology: A Tribute to Julius Axelrod.* Professor Snyder was a research associate with Dr. Axelrod at the National Institutes of Health.

**Barry L. Jacobs,** Ph.D., is currently a professor in the program of neuroscience at Princeton University. Professor Jacobs is author of *Serotonin Neurotransmission and Behavior* and *Hallucinogens: Neurochemical, Behavioral and Clinical Perspectives.* He has written many journal articles in the field of neuroscience and contributed numerous chapters to books on behavior and brain science. He has been a member of several panels of the National Institute of Mental Health.

**Joann Ellison Rodgers,** M.S. (Columbia), became Deputy Director of Public Affairs and Director of Media Relations for the Johns Hopkins Medical Institutions in Baltimore, Maryland, in 1984 after 18 years as an award-winning science journalist and widely read columnist for the Hearst newspapers.

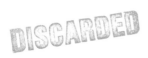